"A deeply moving and essential exploration of facing death in frontline emergency care. This book gives voice to unspoken emotional experiences of healthcare professionals, offering a deeply human perspective of loss, resilience, and meaning making in the Emergency Department. It challenges us to reconsider how we support those who care for others in their most vulnerable moments. A must-read for anyone interested in the intersection of medicine, humanity and ethics."

– **Alison Ross**, *Head of Patient Experience (RN), University Hospital Southampton, United Kingdom*

"This book offers an emotionally resonant and academically rigorous exploration of healthcare professionals' experiences with death in Emergency Departments. Dr Laszlo Penzes brings rare insight, drawing on both scholarly research and lived experience, to illuminate the ethical, cultural, and human dimensions of end-of-life encounters in high-pressure clinical settings. Essential reading for anyone interested in the intersection of emergency care, professional identity, and the human condition."

– **James Wilson**, *Senior Lecturer in Nursing, University of Chichester, United Kingdom*

"This concise and deeply human book explores the emotional, psychological, and moral toll of experiencing death in the Emergency Department. Bridging the gap between scientific palliative care literature and the self-help grief genre, it challenges readers to consider the hidden cost of care and the resilience required to carry on after delivering the worst news imaginable. A must read for all professionals working in emergency care."

– **Prof Julian Kause**, *Professor of Medicine, RCSI Medical University, Bahrain*

"This book is an authentic, thought-provoking portrayal of what it means to care for others while confronting one's own limits. It sheds light on the cultural complexities, social disconnection, and spiritual needs that emerge at the end of life. Ideal for readers who believe that effective healthcare begins with compassion and cultural respect."

– **Dr Matsikachando Moyo**, *Lecturer in Social Sciences and Nursing, Southampton Solent University, United Kingdom*

Experiencing Death in the Emergency Department

This book draws on original research to illuminate how the personal values and norms of healthcare professionals in the Emergency Department (ED) influence how they experience the death of a patient, and develop tools and strategies to cope with these experiences. Experiencing death in the ED begins by considering the nature of death in the ED; rather than planned and dignified, as part of a palliative or end-of-life care pathway, it is often abrupt and unexpected. Healthcare practitioners can be expected to 'move on' and function almost immediately after a death in this busy work environment, carrying the potential for emotional distress and psychological trauma.

Penzes investigates the psychological, emotional, social, and spiritual dimensions of death and how it influences the lives of those people who are directly involved, including the healthcare professionals looking after their patients. Presenting models of bereavement, he looks specifically at deaths in the ED, exploring what makes a death memorable, and how the patient can be objectified or humanised. A discussion of how the personal values and norms of practitioners help them to make sense of deaths they've experienced is followed up with an exploration of the emotional labour of death and its impact on healthcare professionals' behaviours, decisions, and priorities, influencing their coping mechanisms, the care provided for other patients, and even their career choices.

Arguing that developing emotional intelligence, self-awareness, and effective self-management of personal values is crucial in providing holistic care to patients and their families, this book is an important read for researchers and students from nursing, medicine, allied health, business studies, and sociology. It is of particular value for those with an interest in grief and bereavement, trauma, workforce development and wellbeing, and emergency care nursing.

Dr Laszlo Penzes is a trained emergency nurse, researcher, former lecturer, and public and motivational speaker, with a doctorate in Health Sciences, working as senior education manager at one of the largest ambulance service trusts in Southern England. Research interests include emergency medicine, end-of-life care, emotional intelligence, psychology, and human factors in communication and learning.

Routledge Research in Nursing and Midwifery

Substance Use, End of Life Care and Multiple Deprivation
Practice and Research
Edited by Gary Witham, Sarah Galvani, Sam Wright and Gemma A. Yarwood

Nursing a Radical Imagination
Moving from Theory and History to Action and Alternate Futures
Edited by Jess Dillard-Wright, Jane Hopkins-Walsh, and Brandon Brown

Researching Racism in Nursing
Reflexive Accounts and Personal Stories
Edited by Helen Allan and Michael Traynor

Caring in Context
An Ethnography of Cancer Nursing in India
Virgina LeBaron

The Contested Space of Birth
What Makes a Good Birth?
Edited by Nicole Thualagant and Katja Schroder

For more information about this series, please visit: https://www.routledge.com/Routledge-Research-in-Nursing/book-series/RRIN

Experiencing Death in the Emergency Department

How Healthcare Professionals Experience, Make Sense of, and are Influenced by, Death and Dying

Laszlo Penzes

Routledge
Taylor & Francis Group
LONDON AND NEW YORK

First published 2026
by Routledge
4 Park Square, Milton Park, Abingdon, Oxon OX14 4RN

and by Routledge
605 Third Avenue, New York, NY 10158

Routledge is an imprint of the Taylor & Francis Group, an informa business

British Library Cataloguing-in-Publication Data
A catalogue record for this book is available from the British Library

ISBN: 9781032660899 (hbk)
ISBN: 9781032661711 (pbk)
ISBN: 9781032660912 (ebk)

DOI: 10.4324/9781032660912

Typeset in Times New Roman
by codeMantra

To all healthcare professionals, who put on the line often their own wellbeing, mental and physical health, to save their patients' lives, improve their condition, and support their families, if they must face the inevitable or unimaginable.

Contents

Figures

Tables

About the author

Dr Laszlo Penzes is a trained emergency nurse, researcher, former lecturer, and public and motivational speaker, with a doctorate in Health Sciences, working as senior education manager at one of the largest ambulance service trusts in Southern England. Research interests include emergency medicine, end-of-life care, emotional intelligence, psychology, and human factors in communication and learning.

Foreword

In this world, nothing is certain, except death and taxes.

The commonly known phrase, attributed to the American statesman Benjamin Franklin, as part of a letter written in the late 1700s, suggests that there are certainties in life, shared by humans universally, which simply can't be avoided.

Death is one of them.

Death as a discussion topic in the Western culture was an uncomfortable subject for decades. The advancement of palliative and end-of-life care had a significant role in breaking this taboo and helped us better understand and prepare for this inevitable event. Beyond understanding the impact on patients and their families, exploring the influence on those caring for the dying or grieving became the focal point of numerous research studies, investigating this phenomenon. While we understand more profoundly the physical, psychological, and emotional toll this experience has on healthcare professionals (HCPs), this book will uncover how personal values, rooted in our upbringing, our cultural and social background, our faith or spiritual beliefs, the norms of our profession and organisation we work for, and the society we live in define how we make sense, cope, learn from, and live with the death experience. My motivation for conducting the research this book is based on had not only a professional, but also a very personal aspect.

I almost lost my life in the process.

Before sharing details of this personal perspective, let me reveal how my professional curiosity about this subject unfolded over the years, while working as a nurse. The death experience was known to me, as I have encountered deaths in my own family, yet this has become a more frequent experience during my nursing student years. As a student, during my practice placements, I have experienced death in clinical settings, in multiple forms and a wide variety of environments. One of my placements was in a palliative care hospice, where patients and families, knowing about the approach of the inevitable, were expecting death to happen every single day. Even in this environment, death often was unexpected, when it arrived sooner than some might have thought. However, this was the environment where I have learned to focus on the 'bright side' of the experience, to celebrate the happy moments of a life often lived to the full, and the significant role of dignity. I remember how one morning a patient took her last breath right in front me, while doing cardiovascular observations. Yet this is where I have learned the difficulty of maintaining a fragile balance between remaining human and letting being affected by the experience and wearing 'an armour and a shield', to be able to carry on with the everyday nursing duties.

Death on a hospital ward was slightly different. Seeing a patient for weeks, establishing a rapport, building a good relationship with the family, and then coming to work one morning to hear that the patient died overnight often had personal effect on me. It felt like losing a family member or a friend. Seeing death while nursing in the community brought to the surface again different emotions. I remember once when I had to visit a patient for the first time, early in the morning and I found her dead-on-arrival. Having to establish that the patient has truly no signs of life, in an empty house, as a student, felt very daunting at that time. Soon after starting my nursing career in the Emergency Department (ED), I quickly understood that death in this environment is different from anything else that I have experienced before. My exposure to death events in the ED environment was often not only more frequent, but the nature and characteristics of these deaths felt more traumatic and unexpected compared to any other clinical area I have worked in as a student nurse. Reflecting on my own firsthand experiences and having countless informal conversations with colleagues, I have noticed that there can be significant differences in how ED staff may manage and cope with these events. This led me to be interested in understanding why and how people have different reactions to the same traumatic event and how they are affected by it, in the short and long term. I have also become extremely interested in the coping strategies that clinical staff may adopt and which of these prove to be successful and sustainable.

In April 2020, whilst working as a member of staff in the ED of my local acute hospital, I got infected with COVID-19. I was halfway through the six-year period of conducting my research and completing my doctorate. At that time, I was in my mid-forties, healthy, with no pre-existing medical conditions. Yet, after being confirmed positive for COVID-19 my physical condition has declined so quickly and dramatically that I was taken with the ambulance into my own workplace. Becoming a patient where you come to work daily, your fellow colleagues treating and looking after you, felt almost unreal. The same day I became an inpatient in intensive care and placed on non-invasive ventilation. As the treatment was not helping, two days later I gave consent to be put under general anaesthetic in an induced coma and be connected to life-supporting equipment. Few days later my wife was told that in a final attempt to improve my condition, and at that point save my life, I will be transported to London for an ECMO (Extra-Corporal Membrane Oxygenation) treatment. The medical prognosis of surviving the intervention was 40%.

40%. The odds were not in my favour.

Amid the greatest health threat of our generation, which according to the World Health Organization (WHO) (2021), in 2020 alone caused the death of an estimated 3 million people worldwide, I had a greater chance to leave the hospital in a body bag, instead of on my own feet. However, as you can guess, by the simple fact that you are reading this book, my story had a happy ending. My healing and later my recovery was so quick, being discharged after spending a month in two hospitals, that the medical team and later the national and international media who picked up my story was referring to me as the 'miracle man'.

Part of me wishes, I should have never gone through this terrifying experience. If I had a choice, I would spare my family, friends, colleagues, neighbours, everyone I care about from all the pain, worries, desperation, and sleepless nights they had to go through. However, I must admit, I admire their faith, strength, and perseverance they showed when I was at my worst. They have never given up on me; they were always ready to welcome me home again; they never let their hope die. Deep down I know, besides modern medical equipment, clinical knowledge and expertise of all the doctors involved in my treatment, exceptional patient care of all the nurses, and healthcare assistants looking after me, the fact that I'm alive and well is also because of the thoughts, prayers, love, and support offered by so many. Yet my other part does not regret this experience, as it changed me. It changed the way I see myself, the people I love, and the world surrounding me. This near-death experience added an additional impetus to explore the topic of death experiences in the ED, especially in the light of personal values and norms influencing individual experiences.

HCPs' experiences of death during the height of the pandemic were often described as unprecedented. There were a greater number of deaths in the ED during this period, and often these deaths were traumatic and sudden. Difficulties were exacerbated by visiting restrictions being in place, putting an even greater psychological and emotional pressure on frontline workers due to the lack of support from families. The direct involvement of healthcare professionals in the diagnosis, treatment, and care of patients with COVID-19, associated with a high mortality rate, has taken a toll on their physical, mental, and emotional wellbeing. Numerous studies suggest that exposure of HCPs to COVID-19 cases is associated with a higher risk of symptoms of depression, post-traumatic stress disorder, and other mental health issues (Cadogan and Hughes, 2021; Shanafelt et al., 2020; Erdem and Lucey, 2021; Jaiswal et al., 2020). It is important to state all the above, as the data collection and analysis of the research study this book is based on, happened during the COVID-19 pandemic in 2021, some of the stories and experiences shared by participants during the interviews, relating directly to deaths caused by this disease.

While ED remains a place with its main purpose to save lives and improve clinical conditions, caring for the dying and managing the consequences of witnessing death by HCPs remains a priority without any doubt. Personal values and norms will influence HCP's attitudes towards death, impacting their decisions, priorities, and behaviours in their personal and professional life. My aim, through this book, is to raise awareness about this issue, articulate the need for further work to inform practice, and contribute to a better preparedness for such potentially traumatic events.

Reference list

Cadogan, C.A., Hughes, C.M. (2021). On the frontline against COVID-19: Community pharmacists' contribution during a public health crisis. *Research in Social and Administrative Pharmacy*, 17(1), pp. 2032–2035.

Erdem, H., Lucey, D.R. (2021). Healthcare worker infections and deaths due to COVID-19: A survey from 37 nations and a call for WHO to post national data on their website. *International Journal of Infectious Diseases*, 102, pp. 239–241.

Jaiswal, A., Singh, T., Arya, Y.K. (2020). "Psychological Antibodies" to safeguard frontline healthcare warriors mental health against COVID-19 pandemic-related psychopathology. *Frontiers in Psychiatry*, 2020(11), p. 590160. Available at: https://www.frontiersin.org/articles/10.3389/fpsyt.2020.590160/full (Accessed: 12 April 2024).

Shanafelt, T., Ripp, J., Trockel, M. (2020). Understanding and addressing sources of anxiety among health care professionals during the COVID-19 pandemic. *Journal of American Medical Association,* 323(21), pp. 2133–2134.

World Health Organisation (2021). *The true death toll of COVID-19. Estimating global excess mortality.* Available at: https://www.who.int/data/stories/the-true-death-toll-of-covid-19-estimating-global-excess-mortality (Accessed: 10 February 2025).

Preface
Healthcare Professionals Grading in the United Kingdom

Band 1 – Support Worker (phased out)

- **Role**: Basic support tasks (e.g., portering, cleaning)
- **Note**: Largely phased out; most roles now start at Band 2

Band 2 – Healthcare Assistant (HCA)

- **Role**: Personal care (washing, feeding, toileting), basic observations
- **Setting**: Hospitals, care homes, community

Band 3 – Senior HCA/Clinical Support Worker

- **Role**: More advanced clinical tasks (e.g., ECGs, wound care), some supervision
- **Often**: A stepping stone to nursing training

Band 4 – Assistant Practitioner/Nursing Associate

- **Role**: Bridge between HCAs and registered nurses
- **Duties**: Clinical tasks under registered nurse supervision, some patient assessments

Band 5 – Registered Nurse/Staff Nurse

- **Role**: Fully qualified nurse (adult, child, mental health, learning disability)
- **Duties**: Patient care planning, medication administration, clinical decision-making

Band 6 – Sister/Charge Nurse/Specialist Nurse

- **Role**: Experienced nurse often with specialist skills (e.g., diabetes, tissue viability)
- **Duties**: Leadership, mentoring, complex care management

Band 7 – Senior Sister/Senior Charge Nurse/Ward Manager/Advanced Clinical Practitioner

- **Role**: Advanced clinical practice or team leadership
- **Duties**: Service development, staff management, high-level clinical expertise

Band 8a–8d – Nurse Consultant/Senior Management

- **Role**: Strategic leadership, service redesign, clinical governance
- **Includes:**
    - 8a: Matron, Clinical Nurse Specialist
    - 8b–8d: Heads of Nursing, Nurse Consultants, Directors

Foundation Training (Junior Doctors)

- **FY1 (Foundation Year 1)**
    - **Role**: Newly qualified doctor under close supervision
    - **Duties**: Basic clinical tasks, patient reviews, documentation
- **FY2 (Foundation Year 2)**
    - **Role**: More independent practice
    - **Duties**: Greater responsibility, on-call shifts, prescribing

Specialty Training (ST)/Core Training (CT)

- **CT1–CT3/ST1–ST3**
    - **Role**: Early specialty training (e.g., GP, surgery, medicine)
    - **Duties**: Developing specialty-specific skills, supervised procedures
- **ST4–ST8 (Higher Specialty Training – including Registrar)**
    - **Role**: Advanced training in chosen specialty
    - **Duties**: Leading ward rounds, complex procedures, teaching juniors

Specialty Doctor/Specialist Grade

- **Specialty Doctor**
    - **Role**: Experienced non-training doctor
    - **Duties**: Independent practice, often long-term in one specialty
- **Specialist Grade**
    - **Role**: Senior non-consultant with high expertise
    - **Duties**: Advanced clinical work, leadership, supervision

Consultant

- **Role**: Senior doctor with full responsibility for patient care
- **Duties**: Clinical leadership, service development, teaching, research

General Practitioner (GP)

- **Role**: Primary care; employed by a GP practice or NHS organisation

Acknowledgements

I would like to thank my family, my wife, and two boys, who learned how to cope with my absence, while spending my weekends researching and writing. I am speechless, when I think of their resilience and bravery while I was fighting for my life, during the COVID-19 pandemic, and for their gentle encouragement, not to give up, but continue my research, after this life-changing event.

I am thankful for my research supervisors Dr Michelle Myall and Dr Joanne Turnbull, who always empathised with my struggles, but pushed me beyond my limits, to witness how I gain integrity, creativity, and resilience in the process. I also appreciate all the support I've received from my former supervisors Prof Catherine Pope and Prof Robert Crouch who always believed in me, Robert also acting as a clinical advisor, helping me better understand the realities of Emergency Services.

My gratitude also goes for all the participants of my research study, who allowed me to have a glimpse of their thoughts and feelings, offering me the chance to know some remarkable humans working in the frontline of our healthcare system. Countless number of friends, work colleagues, PhD students, former lecturers, and tutors played a significant role in inspiring and supporting me.

I am also thankful for the more mature and empathetic person that I've become during the process of researching, and then writing this book.

Abbreviations

ARC	Applied Research Collaboration
COVID-19	Coronavirus Disease 2019
CPR	Cardio-Pulmonary Resuscitation
CT	Computed tomography
ECMO	Extra-Corporal Membrane Oxygenation
ED	Emergency Department
EEG	Electroencephalogram
HCP	Healthcare Professional
IPA	Interpretative Phenomenological Analysis
MRI	Magnetic Resonance Imaging
NHS	National Health Services (UK)
NICE	The National Institute for Health and Care Excellence (UK)
NIHR	National Institute for Health and Care Research (UK)
NMC	Nursing and Midwifery Council (UK)
PTSD	Post-Traumatic Stress Disorder
RCN	Royal College of Nursing (UK)
TRIM	Trauma Risk Assessment
UK	United Kingdom
US(A)	United States (of America)
WHO	World Health Organization

Chapter 1

Introduction

Imagine for a moment that you are a nurse or a doctor working in the Emergency Department (ED). During one of your shifts an 18-year-old girl is brought in with severe injuries sustained from a road traffic accident, being hit by a drunk driver, while cycling home. Despite all your efforts to save her life, she dies in the department. Her parents are waiting outside, and you are just about to meet them and deliver the unimaginable news, that she will never return home.

Now imagine experiencing something similar two or three times in a week.

Death in the ED is different compared to other clinical areas, not only because of its frequency, but mostly because of its nature, often being traumatic, sudden, or unexpected. Healthcare professionals (HCPs) will experience death as part of their daily work, through the lenses of their personal values. Unlike taking off their civilian clothes and changing into their uniform at the beginning of a shift, personal values are not something that they could lightly step in and out, as it's bonded in their identity, defining the way they see themselves and the world around us.

The importance of studying the influence of the death experience

Human life is unique, irreplaceable, and fragile, and death is an inevitable stage of this life. While in a clinical environment there might be a tendency to look at the end of someone's life as a natural, biological process, death may have psychological, emotional, social, and spiritual dimensions (Mierendorf and Gidvani, 2014), having an influence on the lives of people who are directly involved, including the HCPs looking after their patients (Iserson, 2000). While death can be planned and dignified, as part of a palliative or end-of-life care pathway, at home, in a hospice, or even in a hospital ward, death in the ED is often a sudden and unexpected event (Mierendorf and Gidvani, 2014).

The National Health Service (NHS) Long-Term Plan (NHS England, 2019) aims to reduce the number of avoidable emergency admissions in the last year of a person's life; however, recent statistics shows that these present an increasing tendency for the past ten years in England (Nuffield Trust, 2022). While the proportion of deaths that occur in a hospital setting has decreased from 51% in 2011 to 44% in

DOI: 10.4324/9781032660912-1

2021, with deaths occurring at home during the COVID-19 pandemic being above the previous five-year average (Nuffield Trust, 2020), the proportion of three or more emergency admissions in the last year of a person's life increased from 21% in 2009 to 25% in 2018 (Nuffield Trust, 2022).

What makes the experience in the ED so different?

The ED is a 'front door' for hospitals, intended for easy access of patients in emergent situations, its culture being defined as 'rescue-oriented', death being perceived as mostly preventable (Kongsuwan et al., 2016). Yet, when death still occurs in the ED, it is still mostly associated with traumatic, unexpected, and sudden deaths, while gradually becomes the referral site for patients with long-term and terminal health problems, seeking symptom control, medical advice, and adequate end-of-life care support (Moller, 2004; Bailey et al., 2011). ED is designed for the rapid cycle of diagnosis-treatment-referral or discharge, with HCPs trained for resuscitation and prioritising life-saving treatments (Marck et al., 2014). As often there is no relationship established between HCPs and the patient, prior of arriving to the ED, deaths that are likely to be perceived as sudden, and as such, challenging and complex, while HCPs are expected to 'move on' and function almost immediately after a death experience in this busy work environment, carrying the potential for emotional distress and psychological trauma (Heiner and Trabulsy, 2011; Jackson et al., 2005). On the contrary, another argument is that emergency nurses have developed coping mechanisms to manage unexpected deaths, through the 'objectification' of the patient, while such mechanisms don't exist with patients dying progressively, posing a greater emotional labour when caring for such patients and their grieving families (Bailey et al., 2011). Either way, HCPs' exposure to the death of their patients can make them conscious of their own mortality, often leading to the development of 'death anxiety', described as a feeling of dread or unease, negatively affecting the quality of care provided to dying patients and their families (Deffner and Bell, 2005).

The emotional and psychological impact and influence on HCPs, of deaths occurring in the ED, are widely researched, together with some of the ethical conflicts these HCPs encounter while looking after the dying patients (Cioffi, 2000; Baird et al., 2014; Sandman and Nordmark, 2006). HCPs working in the ED often find themselves in situations when certain complex decision needs to be made, based not only on medical or nursing considerations, but also accounting for the ethical, moral, legal, anthropological, and philosophical aspects (Petty et al., 2013). Several studies also suggest that care for the dying and attitudes towards death are often influenced by cultural, social, and philosophical belief systems, religious faith, or frequency of exposure to death (Beckstrand et al., 2008; Heaston et al., 2006; Chan, 2004; Peters et al., 2013; Yingting et al., 2018). Yet, the relationship between the personal values and norms held by HCPs, and the experience of death in the ED is under-researched, remaining an area that we just gradually start to understand.

Why personal values and norms matter?

Personal values and norms are "broad desirable goals that motivate people's actions and serve as guiding principles in their lives", some values being more visible than others, expressed through our words, actions, and behaviours (Sagiv et al., 2017). While values define an overall ideal, also shaping the person we are aiming to become in the future, norms are action-oriented 'rules' or 'guides', specifying what needs to be done to achieve this ideal (Parks-Leduc et al., 2015). Some values represent a rule of conduct, such as religious beliefs, while others tend to adapt and change depending on what the individual aims to achieve or become, but ultimately values become part of our personality (Ponizovskiy et al., 2019). As such, they become the main drivers for our actions, aid decision-making or help navigate through difficult situations in our personal and professional life (Parks-Leduc et al., 2015). Values and norms are different for every individual, with some commonalities, and will be usually influenced by a series of factors, such as the cultural and social background, the personal upbringing, shared moral and ethical principles within the social circle, spiritual beliefs, faith, education, career, or self-identity (Gamage et al., 2021). Personal values and norms are bonded in our identity, and play a crucial role when HCPs are experiencing and making sense of death and dying in the ED, influencing the provision of care for other patients, their coping mechanisms or often even their career choices.

Data collection for the research study

The aim of the research study this book is based on, can be summarised in two core objectives:

- To understand how lived experiences of death in the ED are influenced by HCPs personal, cultural, social, spiritual, and moral values and norms.
- To explore the views of HCPs on managing, accessing support, coping with, and preparing for experiences of death in the ED.

As this study sought to examine the views, beliefs, and experiences of people from their own perspective, a qualitative research approach was chosen (Creswell, 2007). Qualitative research was the most appropriate, as it focuses on the meaning of how people make sense of their own lives, experiences, and their structures of the world (Flick, 2010). Qualitative research is interpretative, and I was interested in process, meaning, and understanding gained through words, building abstractions, concepts, and hypotheses from details (Creswell, 2007). The benefits of qualitative research include an in-depth, contextually based, and flexible analysis, while the major challenges could include a higher exposure to bias through personal views and interpretations (Pope and Mays, 2006). My chosen methodology to conduct the study was interpretative phenomenological analysis (IPA), an approach to qualitative research with a particularly psychological perspective on how people make sense of their experience, their personal and social world (Smith and Osborn, 2003 Larkin and Thompson, 2012). An IPA study seeks to understand the meanings of particular experiences, events, and states, characteristic for the participants of the study, by collecting detailed, reflective, first-person accounts from research participants and requires a very detailed examination of the participant's world, also including the invisible aspects of the self, such as the meaning behind the words (Biggerstaff and Thompson, 2008). As opposed to attempts to produce an objective statement of an object or event itself, IPA is concerned with the personal experience of the individual and attempts to discover its personal perception or account of that object or event (Harre, 2004). The outcome of a successful IPA study is interested in 'giving voice' and 'making sense' of a phenomenon. While 'giving voice' can be described as capturing and reflecting upon views, emotions, and concerns of the participants, 'making sense' relates to the interpretation of this experience, often using psychological concepts to extend beyond their direct meaning (Larkin et al., 2006).

Initially data collection was designed to use face-to-face semi-structured interviews with a small group of participants. In March 2020, new restrictions and limitations were introduced as a response to the COVID-19 pandemic across all healthcare institutions in England. As a mitigation measure and to adhere to the social distancing and infection prevention measures of the acute hospital where the study was conducted, interviews were completed using a secure, online video-calling platform. Interviews were in average 60-minute long, to allow an in-depth conversation, audio-recorded, then transcribed and analysed. Participants comprised of HCPs recruited from the same ED of a large NHS Foundation Trust Hospital in Southern England. This is a 57-bed unit, divided into seven sections, including the Major Injuries Unit and Initial Assessment, Ambulatory Majors, Resuscitation Room, Minor Injury Unit, Clinical Decision Unit one and two, and an Enhanced Care Suite. The unit has a rapid turnover of patients over the age of 17 who usually stay in the department for less than ten hours. The ED has a sub-unit dedicated for paediatric patients. The number of clinical staff working within the department at the time of the study was approximately 150. Participants were purposively selected to give diversity in terms of profession, gender, age, nationality, and work experience in the ED, to capture different perspectives in understanding the experiences of death. Seven of the participants were nurses, working in Band 5, 6, and 7 roles; five were doctors, of which one was a junior doctor, two were registrars, and two were consultants; three were healthcare assistants and healthcare support workers, and the remaining two were advanced clinical practitioners. The number of male and female participants was almost equal, mostly represented by the 20–39 age group, five working for more than ten years in the ED, eight between six and ten years, while four of them between one and five years. Characteristics of the study participants who took part in the interviews are listed in Table 1.1.

As this book will feature a series of direct quotes, any information identifying the study participants, individuals, or the hospital where the study was conducted, were removed. Participants are referred to in this book using pseudonyms

Table 1.1 Characteristics of the study participants

Profession/role				
Healthcare assistant	*Nurse*	*Advanced clinical practitioner*	*Doctor*	*Total*
3	7	2	5	17
Gender				
Female	*Male*		*Total*	
8	9		17	
Age				
20–29	*30–39*	*40–49*	*Total*	
6	7	4	17	
Experience in the ED				
1–5 years	*6–10 years*	*10+ years*	*Total*	
4	8	5	17	
Leadership				
Leadership role	*Non-leadership role*		*Total*	
12	5		17	
Nurses professional band				
Band 5	*Band 6*	*Band 7*	*Total*	
1	3	3	7	
Doctors professional grade				
Junior	*Registrar*	*Consultant*	*Total*	
1	2	2	5	
Healthcare assistant professional band				
Band 2	*Band 3*		*Total*	
2	1		3	

alongside their real job role, which serve the purpose of protecting their identity and maintain confidentiality.

Structure of this book

This book will start by exploring the phenomenon of 'ageing population' across the developed Western societies, and how people dying in an acute hospital has become a more frequent occurrence compared to other societies. This will be followed by an analysis of how greater expectation from patients about response time and level of treatment, has increased the number of attendances at the ED, inevitably increasing the risk of mortality in this environment. Dying in a clinical environment is a complex issue encountered daily by HCPs, as they may have developed a close relationship with their patients and their families, creating a sense of grief, provoking strong physiological, psychological, or emotional responses. HCPs experiences of death in the ED will often incorporate their interaction, relationship, communication, connection with their patients and their families, including the treatment and the care provided for the dying.

Understanding death beyond the biological dimension, will start with exploring the social aspect of death, describing how social death builds certain activities around a patient in a hospital, how institutionalisation of death creates a detachment from social activities, HCPs often treating progressively dying patients as being already dead. The cultural aspect of death will be discussed next, acknowledging how the Western concept of death is different from those in some other cultures, including cultures dominated by the views of different religions, how these cultures developed different ways to cope with death, creating often barriers and discomfort in HCPs, when it comes to providing culturally sensitive end-of-life care. The spiritual aspect of death will explore how spirituality means more than simply religious beliefs, defining individual's search for purpose in life and meaning in death, how dying patients often experience an existential suffering, and how HCPs can assist patients nearing death to alleviate death anxiety. The discussion will continue with the role of moral values in HCP's care for their dying patients and how moral reasoning supports HCPs to treat their patients with dignity and respect. The complexity of the bereavement process and various models of grieving will be then explored.

The findings of my research study will be discussed in the following three consecutive chapters, starting with how HCPs experience death in the ED, what makes a death 'more memorable' than others and how patients are often first objectified, only to be humanised again, as part of this experience. Understanding how HCPs are making sense of the death experience will be discussed through exploring what kind of meaning they find in this experience, how this aligns with their personal, institutional, or societal values, and finally how faith, and spiritual or religious beliefs influence this search for meaning. The influence that the death experience has on HCPs in their professional and personal life, how that affects aspects such as patient care or even career decisions, will conclude our discussion, including a few recommendations for practice and further research.

Death is a difficult discussion topic. You know it when a 'veteran' consultant with decades of emergency and critical care experience, that kind of persona that seems 'untouchable' from the outside, suddenly breaks in tears in the middle of the participant interview, when recalling some of the challenging cases, that will probably live with him forever. Experiencing death and researching the influence of this experience on my fellow frontline workers, has certainly changed me, making me a more mature and empathetic professional and human, to whom life is a unique, irreplaceable, precious gift, worth protecting and cherishing.

Reference list

Bailey, C., Murphy, R., Porock, D. (2011). Dying cases in emergency places: Caring for the dying in Emergency Departments. *Social Science and Medicine*, 73(9), pp. 1371–1377.

Baird, G., Sammy, I., Nunes, P., Paul, J. (2014). Attitudes and practices regarding resuscitation in Emergency Departments in Trinidad and Tobago. *Emergency Medicine Journal*, 31(11), pp. 889–893.

Beckstrand, R., Smith, M.D., Heaston, S., Bond, A.E. (2008). Emergency nurses' perceptions of size, frequency, and magnitude of obstacles and supportive behaviours in end-of-life care. *Journal of Emergency Nursing*, 34(3), pp. 290–300.

Biggerstaff, D., Thompson, A.R. (2008). Interpretative phenomenological analysis (IPA): A qualitative methodology of choice in healthcare research. *Qualitative Research in Psychology*, 5(3), pp. 214–224.

Chan, G.K. (2004). End-of-life models and Emergency Department care. *Academic Emergency Medicine*, 11(1), pp. 79–86.

Cioffi, J. (2000). Nurses' experiences of making decisions to call emergency assistance to their patients. *Journal of Advanced Nursing*, 32(1), pp. 108–114.

Creswell, J.W. (2007). *Qualitative inquiry and research design: Choosing among five approaches* (2nd Edition). London: Sage.

Deffner, J.M., Bell, S.K. (2005). Nurses' death anxiety, comfort level during communication with patients and families regarding death, and exposure to communication education: A quantitative study. *Journal of Nurses in Staff Development*, 21(1), pp. 19–23.

Flick, U. (2010). *An introduction to qualitative research* (4th Edition). New Delhi: Sage Publication.

Gamage, K.A., Dehideniya, D.M., Ekanayake, S.Y. (2021). The role of personal values in learning approaches and student achievements. *Behavioral Sciences*, 11(7), p. 102.

Harre, R. (2004). Staking our claim for qualitative psychology as science. *Qualitative Research in Psychology*, 1(1), pp. 3–14.

Heaston, S., Beckstrand, R.L., Bond, A.E., Palmer, S.P. (2006). Emergency nurses' perceptions of obstacles and supportive behaviors in end-of-life care. *Journal of Emergency Nursing*, 32(6), pp. 477–485.

Heiner, J.D., Trabulsy, M.E. (2011). Coping with the death of a patient in the Emergency Department. *Annals of Emergency Medicine*, 58(3), pp. 295–298.

Iserson, K.V. (2000). Notifying survivors about sudden, unexpected deaths. *The Western Journal of Medicine*, 173(4), pp. 261–265.

Jackson, V.A., Sullivan, A.M., Gadmer, N.M., Seltzer, D., Mitchell, A.M., Lakoma, M.D., Arnold, R.M., Block, S.D. (2005). "It was haunting…": Physicians' descriptions of emotionally powerful patient deaths. *Academic Medicine*, 80(7), pp. 648–656.

Kongsuwan, W., Matchim, Y., Nilmanat, K., Locsin, R.C., Tanioka, T., Yasuhara, Y. (2016). Lived experience of caring for dying patients in emergency room. *International Nursing Review*, 63(1), pp. 132–138.

Larkin, M., Watts, S., Clifton, E. (2006). Giving voice and making sense in interpretative phenomenological analysis. *Qualitative Research in Psychology*, 3(2), pp. 102–120.

Larkin, M., Thompson, A. (2012). Interpretative phenomenological analysis, in A. Thompson & D. Harper (eds.), *Qualitative research methods in mental health and psychotherapy: A guide for students and practitioners*. Oxford: John Wiley & Sons.

Marck, C.H., Weil, J., Lane, H., Weiland, T.J., Philip, J., Boughey, M., Jelinek, G.A. (2014). Care of the dying cancer patient in the Emergency Department: Findings from a national survey of Australian Emergency Department clinicians. *Internal Medicine Journal*, 44(4), pp. 362–368.

Mierendorf, S.M., Gidvani, V. (2014). Palliative care in the Emergency Department. *The Permanente Journal*, 18(2), pp. 77–85.

Moller, D.W. (2004). *Dancing with broken bones: Portraits of death and dying among inner-city poor*. Oxford and New York: Oxford University Press.

NHS England (2019). *The NHS long-term plan.* Available at: https://www.longtermplan.nhs.uk/wp-content/uploads/2019/08/nhs-long-term-plan-version-1.2.pdf (Accessed: 21 November 2024).

Nuffield Trust (2020). *Chart of the week: Home deaths account for as many excess deaths since start of the pandemic as deaths in care homes*. Available at: https://www.nuffieldtrust.org.uk/resource/home-deaths-now-account-for-as-many-excess-deaths-since-the-start-of-the-pandemic-as-deaths-in-care-homes (Accessed: 09 October 2024).

Nuffield Trust (2022). *End-of-life care. Quality watch indicator.* Available at: https://www.nuffieldtrust.org.uk/resource/end-of-life-care (Accessed: 12 December 2024).

Parks-Leduc, L., Feldman, G., Bardi, A. (2015). Personality traits and personal values: A meta-analysis. *Personality and Social Psychology Review*, 19(1), pp. 3–29.

Peters, L., Cant, R., Payne, S., O'Connor, M., McDermott, F., Hood, K., Morphet, J., Shimoinaba, K. (2013). Emergency and palliative care nurses' levels of anxiety about death and coping with death: A questionnaire survey. *Australasian Emergency Nursing Journal*, 16(4), pp. 152–159.

Petty, K., DeGarmo, N., Aitchison, R. (2013). Ethical considerations in resuscitation. *Disease-a-Month*, 59(5), pp. 217–220.

Ponizovskiy, V., Grigoryan, L., Kühnen, U., Boehnke, K. (2019). Social construction of the value–behavior relation. *Frontiers in Psychology*, 10, p. 934.

Pope, C., Mays, N. (2006). *Qualitative research in health care* (3rd Edition). London: BMJ Books.

Sagiv, L., Roccas, S., Cieciuch, J., Schwartz, S.H. (2017). Personal values in human life. *Nature Human Behaviour*, 1(9), p. 630.

Sandman, L., Nordmark, A. (2006). Ethical conflicts in prehospital emergency care. *Nursing Ethics*, 13(6), pp. 592–607.

Smith, J.A., Osborn, M. (2003). *Qualitative psychology: A practical guide to research methods*. New York: Sage Publications.

Yingting, Z., Yash Pal, R., Wai, T., Wilson, S., Lee, A., Ong, M., Hwaa, T.L. (2018). Spiritual perspectives of emergency medicine doctors and nurses in caring for end-of-life patients: A mixed-method study. *International Emergency Nursing*, 37, pp. 13–22.

Chapter 2

Death and dying in a healthcare setting

A profound understanding of a phenomenon requires an in-depth knowledge of the context and a discovery of the root causes. This is why the first chapter will start by exploring the statistical link between an overall ageing population and the increased number of deaths recorded in a healthcare setting across the Westernised, industrially developed countries. Experiencing death in a hospital environment and more specifically in the Emergency Department (ED), alongside the patient and healthcare professional (HCP) relationship, as a key factor in understanding the lived experiences of death, will also be analysed. This relationship will often incorporate HCP's interaction, relationship, communication, connection with their patients, and their families, including the treatment and care provided for the dying. Various perceptions and interpretations about dignity in the ED will be then discussed, including the importance of the physical environment, and the impact of family and friends being close to the dying patient. This chapter will conclude with discussing the physical, psychological, and emotional influences on HCPs, of the death of their patients.

Ageing and death in numbers

Direct references to official statistics related to deaths in the ED are often difficult to find, as most of the published data relates to the number of deaths in hospitals in general, and not in a specific department. However, to have an estimate of the possible magnitude of this issue, I decided to have a look at the greater picture, including ageing statistics, ED admission, and hospital mortality figures. Statistics suggest that the population of Europe has recorded a significant ageing rate over a period of 20 years, since the mid-nineties. The median age is an indicator that divides a population into two parts of equal size, either older or younger than the median age. In 1996, the median age of the 27 European countries population was 36.8 years, in 2016, the median age recorded was almost six years higher, at 42.6 years. In 2016, the people aged 65 and over, represented 19.2% of the total European population, with a life expectancy of more than 80 years in average and a slight increase in mortality rates over the last four decades (Eurostat, 2017). Similar trends have been recorded in other economically developed countries, such

DOI: 10.4324/9781032660912-2

as the USA (PRB, 2019), Australia (AIHW, 2018), and Japan (SBJ, 2019). The exponential relationship between mortality and age has been confirmed by several studies, suggesting that in the developed countries, over a period of two decades, above the age of 35, ageing and all-cause mortality rates are increasing at the same pace (Luder, 1993; Preston et al., 2001; Salinari and De Santis, 2015).

According to a report published by the National Health Services, there were approximately 9.4 million hospital discharges between 2018 and 2019, across 129 trusts in England, from which 287,000 deaths were recorded, either while in hospital or within 30 days of discharge (NHS England, 2020a). Accidental deaths in Scotland recorded an increase of 7% in 2018 compared to the previous year, with the age group of 85 and over being the most affected (24%). The most common causes for these accidental deaths were related to accidental poisoning representing 46% of total number of accidental deaths, falls representing 38% and transport accidents accounting for 7% (NRS, 2018). Another report suggests that in 2016 almost half of all deaths in England (46.9%) occurred in hospital, a percentage significantly higher compared to the deaths occurring in people's own home, in a care home or hospice (Public Health England, 2018).

Attendances to EDs in England have increased from 19.58 million between 2008 and 2009 to almost 25 million ten years later (NHS England, 2020b). A national survey conducted in England in 2015, found that the relatives of people who died in hospital rated overall quality of care in the last three months of life, significantly worse compared to other settings. Approximately three out of ten (31%) respondents rated care in hospitals as fair or poor, compared to the rate of 21% measured for hospices (ONS, 2015). A comparison of the quality of care in the last three months of life, in hospice and in hospital, is represented by Figure 2.1.

On the contrary, a survey conducted at a major teaching hospital in England in 2018, directed at families of adult patients who died whilst in-patients found that 92% of responders agreed that there was good communication from the team informing them that death was expected and communication between the staff and the dying person was sensitive and appropriate to their situation. The huge proportion of the responders, 95% felt that staff took time to listen, while 89% considered that there was an appropriate amount of privacy involved in care. Relatives who felt strongly that the dying patient was treated with dignity and respect, also appears to be increasing in numbers, compared to the statistics from previous year (UHS, 2018).

Death in the hospital

People dying in an acute hospital is a more frequent occurrence in Western societies compared to other societies, where dying at home is more common (Gomes and Higginson, 2008). A cross-national, population-level study conducted in 14 countries, suggests that 45.7% of the terminally ill patients with chronic-degenerative and oncologic diseases, die in hospital, higher than those dying at home, in hospices or other settings such as residential health facilities or an ambulance (Pivodic et al., 2016). Across Western societies, the proportion of people

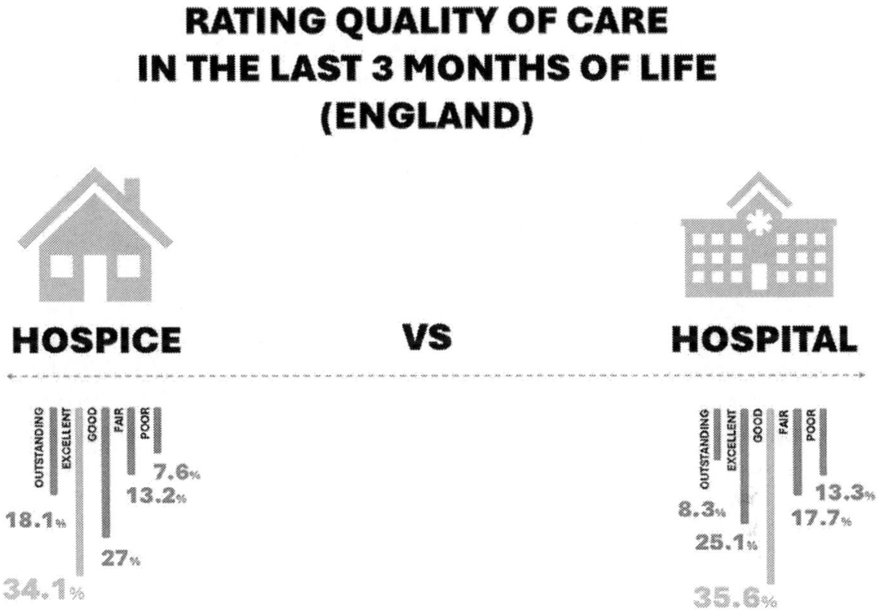

Figure 2.1 Quality of care in the last three months of life in England (adapted from ONS, 2015).

dying at home ranges between 22% and 57%, compared to mainland China, where the proportion of those transferring home to die from critical care units, can be as high as 82%–92% (Lin et al., 2021). This difference is attributed to decisions made on the basis of cultural, religious, and spiritual meanings of the home as a place of death.

The Royal College of Emergency Medicine (2021) has found that at least 4,519 patients died in EDs in England in 2020–2021, during the first waves of COVID-19, numbers being exacerbated by crowding, queuing, and long waits of up to 12 hours of critically ill patients. When nurses and doctors witness the death of their patients in a hospital setting, they might appear to be virtual strangers; however, as providers of care during the last period of their lives, they may have developed a close relationship with them (Aycock & Boyle, 2009). When patients die, HCPs may experience a sense of grief, provoking strong physiological, psychological, or emotional responses, especially if it is unexpected (Newson et al., 2011). A patient's death is being considered one of the most common stressors in a clinical environment, evoking feelings of distress, helplessness, or inadequacy in HCPs; however, often these feelings are not expressed or evaluated (Park et al., 2020). HCPs behaviour when a patient dies, may vary according to the social values, cultural backgrounds, or religious beliefs that they hold, interacting with their perceptions about death (Zheng et al., 2018; Becker et al., 2017). Perceptions can be described as an individual structure of thoughts and feelings about a situation, incorporating previous experiences and memories that help 'making sense' of that situation (McDonald, 2012). Perceptions of death can be a powerful driving force, influencing HCPs' actions and behaviours, influencing their level of death anxiety and provision of supportive end-of-life care (Lai et al., 2018). HCPs that acknowledge and confront their own perceptions of death could potentially offer better provision of end-of-life care in a hospital setting (Hussin et al., 2018; Park et al., 2020).

Death in the Emergency Department

An increasing demand of access to General Practice, and greater expectation from patients about response time and level of treatment, including those on a palliative trajectory, has increased the number of patient attendances at the ED as the first point of contact (Smulowitz et al., 2014; Bailey et al., 2011b). This increase in demand is associated with an increased risk of mortality in the ED, a complex issue encountered daily by clinical staff working in these areas. Patients presenting with chronic disease, acute, rapidly progressing conditions or patients identified as being on a palliative or end-of-life trajectory, historically were usually transferred to a more appropriate setting for treatment or palliation (Pines et al., 2011). However, as healthcare systems more often experience demand that is in excess of staffing levels, these transfers are less likely to be timely (Sanchez et al., 2013). While the ED is not considered an ideal place for palliative care, the culture of emergency medicine is shifting to be more patient goal-centred, from only providing stabilisation of acute medical urgencies, to improve end-of-life care and manage death and dying (Clements et al., 2004; Mierendorf and Gidvani, 2014).

Deaths occurring in the ED still present a range of challenges for HCPs. Emergency doctors could experience an emotional impact during resuscitation, as they can be reminded of the death of a close relative, making death becoming more personal (Kutner and Kilbourn, 2009). During death notification, doctors often experience an impersonal atmosphere, characterised by a busy space, with no well-established doctor–patient relationship and limited time to spend with a bereaved family (Iserson, 2000). Similarly, emergency nurses may also find it difficult to care for dying patients and their families, due the stressful environment, time pressures, lack of space, and a prioritised focus on treatment rather than comfort measures provided for patients (Gerace et al., 2020). Balancing the competing demands of the high-pressure environment of ED, poses one of the greatest challenges for nurses providing end-of-life care in this environment. With critical and acute patients presenting continuously in the ED, often unable to wait for intervention, nurses find it hard to give the dying patients and their families the care, comfort, and attention they deserve (Gerace et al., 2020). Some of the most common obstacles for providing adequate end-of-life care in the ED are detailed in Table 2.1.

Death and the healthcare professional–patient relationship

A traumatic event can be defined as a powerful, extreme, or severe situation, circumstances, or chain of events, able to overwhelm through its intensity a

Table 2.1 Obstacles for end-of-life care provision in the ED

No.	*Common obstacles for end-of-life care in the ED*
1	Time constraints and rapid decision-making
2	Lack of continuity and patient history
3	Communication barriers and cultural dynamics
4	Inadequate training in palliative care
5	Emotional and moral distress
6	Limited resources and support services

person's ability to cope. The inability of a person to cope with such events may result in unusually strong emotional, cognitive, or behavioural reactions (Meichenbaum, 1994). Nursing and medical professions' roles provide numerous occasions to deal with potentially traumatising situations, emergency services being almost constantly confronted with severe injuries, death, suicide, and suffering (Bennett et al., 2005; McFarlane and Bryant, 2007).

A large proportion of HCPs working in the ED, ranging between 82% and 100%, are frequently exposed to work-related traumatic events, often multiple times a week, or in some cases even daily (Donnelly and Siebert, 2009). When traumatising events are affecting the healthcare professional–patient relationship, these will have emotional and psychological consequences on HCPs (Linklater, 2010). The main priority of the healthcare professional–patient relationship is the patient's wellbeing, and this is based on partnership, intimacy, and reciprocity. This relationship can be defined as a series of interactions with the patient's need at the core and communication as a foundation on which this relationship is built (Rosdahl and Kowalski, 2008). These interactions focus on the ideas, feelings, requirements, and priorities of the patient with the purpose of progressively enhancing optimum physical, mental, and emotional wellbeing (Riley, 2012).

Patients will often experience inequality and powerlessness in this relationship, and may feel vulnerable, reliant, and dependent on HCPs (Webb and Holland, 2011). The relationship and communication between nurses and patients' families will have an impact on both sides' wellbeing, but also the quality and outcome of nursing care (Beaudoin and Ouellet, 2018). When families are experiencing sudden death of their loved ones, the way they handle the grieving process and communicate, will have emotional consequences on HCPs too (Loghmani et al., 2014). Reciprocity is a strong element of the nurse–family relationship, with feedback processes occurring often simultaneously, determining the way parties will think, feel, and behave in this relationship (Gerow et al., 2010).

Factors that can undermine this relationship include segregation of the patients into 'spectacular' and 'subtacular' trajectories, HCPs adopting a distancing attitude or often withdrawing completely from it. In contrast, those communicating with end-of-life patients and their families openly, on an empathetic level, about their prognosis, wishes, or preferences, including elements of spiritual care, are more likely to build a relationship characterised by trust. A common concept in defining the quality of a healthcare professional–patient relationship is related to the trajectories a patient can have in the ED, according to a study conducted in the UK (Bailey et al., 2011a). The 'spectacular' trajectory suggests a public display of the end-of-life in the ED, for example, a major trauma patient, where efforts to save their life require additional nurses, doctors, and often a variety of specialities within the hospital. In contrast, the 'subtacular' trajectory, for example, a patient diagnosed with terminal illness, refers to a 'lower status' care, one that does not consume the same attention as the 'spectacular' and does not evoke the heroic, elaborate reaction of its witnesses (Bailey et al., 2011b). One of the most common behaviours displayed by HCPs towards a 'subtacular' patient and their family, was distancing. This behaviour was often expressed by withdrawing from situations and, in some cases, from the nursing profession altogether.

These observed behaviours had often a detrimental effect on the patients' experience, making them feel 'uncared for', 'forgotten about', and 'neglected'. HCPs and the family could have a disagreement upon the trajectory of a terminally ill patient presenting to ED with an imminent possibility of death (Bailey et al., 2011c). A survey and interviews of Australian palliative and emergency nurses suggest that ED nurses can communicate on a warm, empathetic, and emotional level, encourage the discussion of concerns that otherwise might not be revealed openly by their patients and their families, leading to the development of trust and confidence in this relationship (Peters et al., 2013). Nurses often report that an informative and empathetic communication style, adopted towards patients at the end of their life, especially when time is given to ask questions, will encourage a greater understanding and acceptance of the inevitable, also offering physical and mental health benefits by reducing blood pressure, anxiety, depression, or even pain (Peters et al., 2013). Some emergency nurses are seen as experts in providing quality end-of-life care that is supportive to patients and their family, while others avoided getting involved altogether, lacking skills and confidence in providing this particular type of care (Bailey et al., 2011c).

Another study investigating the quality of care and trajectories in the ED of end-of-life patients in Saudi Arabia found that the relationship between HCPs and a patient at the end of their life is influenced by the amount and depth of discussions, exploring what the patient or their family knows about their overall condition and prognosis. Such discussions should occur in a calm setting, with sufficient time allocated for patients and the family, to express concerns, preferences, and deal with the associated emotions, end-of-life conversations never being one-time discussions, but an ongoing collaborative process (Sadler et al., 2020). A considerable proportion of invasive treatments in the ED occur due to a lack of end-of-life care discussions, prior to a patient's emergency admission, who lives with a terminal illness, and is on an end-of-life pathway already. When a palliative or end-of-life patient is taken into the ED, the patient or family may not be in a mental state to process complex information and consider care options. A palliative patient attending the ED should be considered as an opportunity to review the goals of care, involving not only the primary treating teams but also palliative care services, even if this leads to longer stay (Sadler et al., 2020).

A qualitative study, using interviews and observations of HCPs working in an American ED, found that the transition to end-of-life for a patient coming to the ED can occur suddenly and without warning. For example, a patient who arrests in the ED, transition to end-of-life is short, and there might be impossible to apply palliative care principles, so HCPs are constantly trying to understand whether the actual status is going to be the end for a patient or not, and integrate this knowledge into the care given and communication approaches applied (Chan, 2011). HCPs often report that communication with families in the ED can be sometimes confusing, forced, or pressured, complicated by an atmosphere of high stress and crisis, especially if family treatment wishes are incongruent to the chances of success of the requested, such as invasive interventions. Misunderstanding from the family about the role of hospices and the ED, the signs of impending death, or what death actually looks like, raise challenges for HCPs in managing successfully these relationships (Chan, 2011). Another challenge is raising from the relationship with 'frequent flyers', a term that denotes patients who are heavy users of emergency services, where care could be routinised and given lower priority, increasing the chances to not realise in time if the patient is approaching death (Chan, 2011).

An analysis of open-ended responses in an Australian survey of clinical staff in the ED concluded that open and honest communication with dying patients and their families is very important in establishing accurate prognostic information, managing patient and family expectations, dealing with unrealistic expectations in a timely manner and explanations about the inappropriate nature of particular tests and interventions (Giles et al., 2019). ED nurses often suggest that communication with patients and their families should be in a clear, easily understood language, minimising jargon, and tailoring information to individual levels of understanding. Avoiding or delaying difficult conversations would undermine early recognition of patient and family needs, while giving consistent information to patients and their families and nominating one family spokesperson wherever possible to streamline conversations, was noted as being paramount (Giles et al., 2019).

ED doctors frequently encounter difficulties when family members of a dying patient have unrealistic expectations. However, nurses and nursing assistants often find establishing a relationship based on trust with their patients and their families very difficult, when the same doctors do not update them on the patient's situation in time. This often puts the nursing staff in an uncomfortable position of not knowing what to communicate to the patient's family, often anxiously waiting in the waiting room (Di Leo et al., 2019). Yet, HCPs adopting good communication skills with a family are considered factors in conflict resolution surrounding end-of-life care, especially when the family felt they are heard, they can have a voice, and their wishes are considered (Chan, 2011).

A mixed-methods study that investigated the spiritual perspectives of ED doctors and nurses in caring for end-of-life patients in Singapore argues that acknowledging the spiritual needs of these patients will improve the nurse–patient relationship, as this will help patients to express their physical and emotional needs more openly. Being more involved in decisions concerning their end-of-life pathway promotes the idea for patients of a greater control over their own condition (Yingting et al., 2018). HCPs often report that spirituality for them represents more than religion, being rooted in the meaning of life, becoming more important when one experiences life crisis, such as being diagnosed with terminal illness or nearing end-of-life. Empathy, kindness, appropriately sharing of oneself, or offering chaplaincy services, as part of the relationship with the patient at the end of their life has been recognised by ED nurses as a fundamental attribute in providing spiritual care (Yingting et al., 2018). HCPs can have conflicting views about supporting patients to observe their religious beliefs as part of the spiritual care. While some perceive this as something very personal to the patient and would avoid bringing the topic up, others argue that education on the differing views of various religions may help to better accept the individual views of their patients (Yingting et al., 2018).

Managing dignity in the Emergency Department

Perceptions and interpretations of dignity in the process of a dying person in the ED, from the perspective of HCPs, has a multifaceted aspect, according to the emergency nurses and doctors interviewed in two Spanish hospitals, as part of a phenomenological study. Dignity, beyond anything else, is recognised by clinical staff, as a human attribute, something that only a human being is aware of possessing, demanding, or under certain circumstances, losing (Fernandez-Sola et al., 2017). Dignity of a patient is defined by the HCPs working in the ED, as a person having a human quality, where treating someone with dignity is a moral duty to which even life itself must submit. Maintaining the dignity of a dying person in the ED has complex implications for HCPs. ED is not designed and not an ideal place to provide end-of-life care, as a dying person's dignity implies treating them with respect, recognising their value as a person, as well as offering them autonomy and self-esteem (Fernandez-Sola et al., 2017).

Respecting the dignity of terminally ill patients in the ED also reflects sociocultural aspects of death. From this perspective, displacing death and simply incorporating it into a hospital environment surrounded by technical equipment, the dying person is institutionalised, and may experience isolation, desertion of choice, and amplification of suffering, taking away dignity from the dying process (Fernandez-Sola et al., 2017). 'Humanising' a patient is crucial in providing end-of-life care in the ED, as 'technification', the predominant use of technical equipment and methods in patient care, and 'massification', a state where the demand oversized available resources leading to a decline in quality, can depersonalise care. Dignity also incorporates the interaction and respect towards someone encountering situations of extreme vulnerability, such as being at the end of life. Perceiving a person's dignity implies the right to honour, to a good reputation, to one's own image, to intimacy and physical, mental, and emotional integrity (Fernandez-Sola et al., 2017).

In another Spanish study, ED nurses and doctors suggested that an important factor in promoting dignity for palliative patients in the ED is by creating an environment and developing surroundings that reflect decency, respect, decorum, and worthiness. An environment can be improved to reflect dignity, through softening the lighting, moving palliative patients to a quieter and more private space, or facilitating family members and loved ones to be with patients (Mar Díaz-Cortés et al., 2018). Improving the physical environment by redesigning spaces in the ED has a direct connection to increased patient and family satisfaction and an increase in staff confidence and satisfaction (Mar Díaz-Cortés et al., 2018). However, inadequate spaces in the ED used for communicating bad news to patients and their families are perceived by HCPs as a serious breach to dignity requirements. The privacy provided by a simple curtain is not enough, especially when a patient is in extreme pain and distress as noted by a member of the clinical staff in an Italian study, this is something "a human being does not deserve" (Di Leo et al., 2019). Nurses and doctors referred to ED as a place lacking the means to offer proper comfort for patients, but also family members are using spaces that provide neither intimacy for receiving bad news, nor have basic commodities such as chairs or a coffee table (Di Leo et al., 2019).

Nurses participating in a study in Thailand suggested that a peaceful death is possible in the ED where the family, that is typically the main source of spiritual care, is allowed to spend time with their loved one. As one of the participants of this study states:

> A peaceful death in ER (Emergency Room – author's comment), I think, can be possible but it needs a period of time and a place. When the doctor says to stop resuscitating, there should be a place or a room available where the patient's family members or relatives can stay and the dying patients can be with them.
>
> (Kongsuwan et al., 2016)

While care for the dying in the ED orbits around 'prescriptive or routine care', HCPs are unable to provide the appropriate emotional or psychological support for the family, preparing them for their loved one's death, due primarily because they lack competency and confidence in providing spiritual, emotional, or psychological care (Kongsuwan et al., 2016). Lack of time is also described by the emergency nurses as a crucial factor in missing opportunities to provide palliative care in the ED. As palliative care was considered to take a considerable amount of time, it was never prioritised or integrated into the ED procedures, instead end-of-life patients were transferred to other wards or discharged to their homes to die (Kongsuwan et al., 2016).

Dignity for many dying patients in the ED means offering the opportunity for their loved ones to be close to them, to share their fears, feelings, and their anxiety, to resolve any pending issues or to have the chance to say goodbye. Under such circumstances, dying patients in the ED sometimes need contact more than ever with the family, closeness, enough time, someone to listen, and the comfort and peace that creates the ideal setting for accompaniment (Mar Díaz-Cortés et al., 2018). An

Australian study that interviewed ED doctors and nurses reached to similar conclusions, dignity in the ED being seen as a way of caring for patients and their families that encompasses emotional, spiritual, and even religious aspects (Omoya et al., 2022). Maintaining dignity meant maintaining an empathetic attitude, facilitating a dialogue with patients and family members about all topics, including death. Offering comfort to dying patients and re-assurance that they are not viewed as a burden is an integral part of sustaining dignity, while respecting the wishes of a dying patient, could become a voice in a situation in which a dying patient could become voiceless (Omoya et al., 2022). In contrast, a study conducted in the UK argues that the absence of dignity is also captured in situations when palliative patients are accessing emergency services for symptom control or supportive care as death nears. Often such patients in the ED are labelled as being 'out of place', ED not being considered by staff as 'the right place to die', which manifests in an urgency of transferring the patient to a ward, even with the risk of dying enroute (Bailey et al., 2011b).

The physical, mental, and emotional burden of death on healthcare professionals

Experiencing death is often associated with depression and anxiety symptoms, substance use, or other psychiatric disorders (Keyes et al., 2014). Doctors often demonstrate high-stress responses, recording an increase in heart rate and heart-rate variability when breaking bad news in simulated patient encounters (Brown et.al., 2009). A further survey of 150 emergency doctors suggests that many experienced physical responses to patient death, including insomnia (37%) and fatigue (14%), while in terms of emotional responses, they experienced sadness (60%) and disappointment (38%) (Strote et al., 2011). A combination of emotional and biological stress responses can make emergency doctors more susceptible to job dissatisfaction and burnout (Kutner and Kilbourn, 2009).

Nurses in the ED can also be affected by death, especially when being almost permanently exposed to severe injuries, death, suicide, and suffering in their line of work (Adriaenssens et al., 2012). A UK study suggests that levels of death anxiety were similar in hospice and emergency nurses, although one quarter of emergency nurses showed more fear and less acceptance of death than hospice nurses (Payne et al., 1998). This exposure can potentially lead to loss of productivity, due to a change in professional attitude, or can negatively alter the quality of nursing care. Research has shown that emergency nurses report symptoms of PTSD (post-traumatic stress disorder) after professional confrontations with traumatic events, including sleeping difficulties, nightmares, flashbacks, recurrent images and thoughts, irritability and depression, lack of interest in daily life, loss of hope in the future, and loss of concentration (Gates et al., 2011). A further study reported that the three most distressing events ED nurses are repeatedly confronted with are paediatric death, incidents involving children, and dealing with patients' relatives and family (De Clercq et al., 2011).

Emergency nursing is a complex profession, demanding both physically and emotionally. This demand is arising from dealing with complex patient loads in a fast-paced environment, long shifts, often demanding medical staff, and patient's relatives, causing stress for the ED staff (Healy and Tyrrell, 2011). Emergency nurses experiencing such levels of stress can develop over time compassion fatigue and burnout, conditions that can become overwhelming burdens and can cause physical, mental, and emotional health difficulties. Compassion fatigue is a negative result of working with traumatised patients, described as an emotional, physical, and spiritual exhaustion from witnessing other people suffering (Peery, 2010). Burnout, while very similar to compassion fatigue, is associated with feelings of hopelessness and apathy, which, if not addressed, may develop an inability to fulfil the ED job requirements effectively, also having a negative impact on the provision of care (Hooper et al., 2010). Both compassion fatigue and burnout display similar traits, causing an emergency nurse to become depressed, ineffective, detached or even apathetic. These psychological and emotional consequences, on the long term can lead to a radical decrease of morale, work ethic, job satisfaction, absenteeism, and the inability to co-operate as a team with the fellow co-workers. From a professional perspective, these can have an impact on patient satisfaction and may impact staff retention in the ED (Portnoy, 2011).

Various studies analysed and compared variations in the levels of compassion fatigue, compassion satisfaction, and burnout among nurses from a great variety of specialities including intensive care unit, oncology, nephrology, and emergency services. While the findings of these studies suggest that levels of compassion fatigue are similar among the different specialities, there was a notable difference in compassion satisfaction. ED nurses were reporting lower levels of compassion satisfaction compared to the other type of nurses, revealing also a greater risk of burnout in the ED nurses (Whippen and Canellos, 1991; Hooper et al., 2010). A study surveying 132, year 1 foundation doctors, reported that 61% of them witnessed deaths, including death of young patients, death that lacks dignity, or death of a patient where a strong personal relationship pre-exists, where death remains emotionally distressing, triggering strong reactions (Linklater, 2010). These emotional reactions could include, but not limited to stress, guilt, feelings of numbness, and feeling upset. ED doctors specifically report insomnia, fatigue, sadness, and disappointment after facing unexpected deaths (Redinbaugh et al., 2003; Jackson et al., 2005).

One study, surveying 145 emergency doctors, found that 28% revealed they sometimes considered quitting their jobs, 32% looking for another profession, and 14% looking for various means of counselling. Factors that influenced the intensity level of emotional reactions to a death experience included, the age of the patient, cause of death, and presence of the family (Strote et al., 2011). These effects will also be influenced by the level of training and years of experience a doctor has. These findings are in line with another study which compared nurses' death anxiety and confirmed that nurses' emotional distress was lower as age, education, and nursing experience increased. Emotional distress, which can be defined as a feeling of apprehension, solicitude, or dread, when one thinks of the process of ceasing to be, often has personal and professional consequences, especially when linked to death anxiety (Deffner and Bell, 2005).

Reference list

Adriaenssens, J., de Gucht, V., Maes, S. (2012). The impact of traumatic events on emergency room nurses: Findings from a questionnaire survey. *International Journal of Nursing Studies*, 49(11), pp. 1411–1422.

AIHW – Australian Institute for Health and Welfare (2018). *Older Australia at a glance*. Available: https://www.aihw.gov.au/reports/older-people/older-australia-at-a-glance/contents/demographics-of-older-australians (Accessed: 10 February 2024).

Aycock, N., Boyle, D. (2009). Interventions to manage compassion fatigue in oncology nursing. *Clinical Journal of Oncology Nursing*, 13(2), pp. 183–191.

Bailey, C., Murphy, R., Porock, D. (2011a). Trajectories of end-of-life care in the Emergency Department. *Annals of Emergency Medicine*, 57(4), pp. 362–369.

Bailey, C., Murphy, R., Porock, D. (2011b). Dying cases in emergency places: Caring for the dying in Emergency Departments. *Social Science and Medicine*, 73(9), pp. 1371–1377.

Bailey, C., Murphy, R., Porock, D. (2011c). Professional tears: developing emotional intelligence around death and dying in emergency work. *Journal of Clinical Nursing*, 20(23–24), pp. 3364–3372.

Beaudoin, M.A., Ouellet, N. (2018). An exploration of factors influencing nursing practice with families experiencing perinatal loss. *Recherche en soins infirmiers*, 133(2), pp. 58–69.

Becker, C.A., Wright, G., Schmit, K. (2017). Perceptions of dying well and distressing death by acute care nurses. *Applied Nursing Research*, 33(2), pp. 149–154.

Bennett, P., Williams, Y., Page, N., Hood, K., Woollard, M., Vetter, N. (2005). Associations between organizational and incident factors and emotional distress in emergency ambulance personnel. *British Journal of Clinical Psychology*, 44(6–2), pp. 215–226.

Brown, R., Dunn, S., Byrnes, K., Morris, R., Heinrich, P., Shaw, J. (2009). Doctors' stress responses and poor communication performance in simulated bad news consultations. Academic Medicine, 84(11), pp. 1595–1602.

Chan, G.K. (2011). Trajectories of approaching death in the Emergency Department: Clinician narratives of patient transitions to the end of life. *Journal of Pain and Symptom Management*, 42(6), pp. 864–881.

Clements, P.T., DeRanieri, J.T., Vigil, G.J., Benasutti, K.M. (2004). Life after death: Grief therapy after the sudden traumatic death of a family member. *Perspective Psychiatric Care*, 40(4), pp. 149–154.

De Clercq, F., Deheegher, J., Van Hoorde, H. (2011). Frequency of and subjective response to critical incidents in the prediction of PTSD in emergency personnel. *Journal of Traumatic Stress*, 24(1), pp. 133–136.

Deffner, J.M., Bell, S.K. (2005). Nurses' death anxiety, comfort level during communication with patients and families regarding death, and exposure to communication education: A quantitative study. *Journal of Nurses in Staff Development*, 21(1), pp. 19–23.

Di Leo, S., Alquati, S., Autelitano, C., Costantini, M., Martucci, G., De Vincenzo, F., Kuczynska, B., Morini, A., Trabucco, L., Ursicelli, R., Catania, G., Ghirotto, L. (2019). Palliative care in the Emergency Department as seen by providers and users: a qualitative study. *Scandinavian Journal of Trauma, Resuscitation and Emergency Medicine*, 27, p. 88. Available at: https://doi.org/10.1186/s13049-019-0662-y

Donnelly, E., Siebert, D. (2009). Occupational risk factors in the emergency medical services. *Prehospital Disaster Medicine*, 24(5), pp. 422–429.

Eurostat (2017). *People in the EU - Statistics on demographic changes*. Available: https://ec.europa.eu/eurostat/statistics-explained/index.php?title=People_in_the_EU_-_statistics_on_demographic_changes#Further_Eurostat_information (Accessed: 10 February 2024).

Fernandez-Sola, C., Diaz Cortes, M.M., Hernandez-Padilla, J.M., Aranda Torres, C.J., Granero-Molina J. (2017). Defining dignity in end-of-life care in the Emergency Department. *Nursing Ethics*, 24(1), pp. 20–32.

Gates, D., Gillespie, G., Succop, P. (2011). Violence against nurses and its impact on stress and productivity. *Nursing Economics*, 29(2), pp. 59–67.

Gerace, A., Giles, T., Breaden, K., Hammad, K., Drummond, C., Bradley, S.L., Muir-Cochrane, E. (2020). Nurses' perceptions of dealing with death in the Emergency Department. *Collegian*, 28(1), pp. 71–80.

Gerow, L., Conejo, P., Alonzo, A., Davis, N., Rodgers, S., Domian, E.W. (2010). Creating a curtain of protection: Nurses' experiences of grief following patient death. *Journal of Nursing Scholarship*, 42(2), pp. 122–129.

Giles, T.M., Hammad, K., Breaden, K., Drummond, C., Bradley, S.L., Gerace, A., Muir-Cochrane, E. (2019). Nurses' perceptions and experiences of caring for patients who die in the Emergency Department setting. *International Emergency Nursing*, 47, p. 100789. Available at: https://pubmed.ncbi.nlm.nih.gov/31495727

Gomes, B., Higginson, I.J. (2008). Where people die (1974–2030): Past trends, future projections and implications for care. *Palliative Medicine*, 2008(22), pp. 33–41.

Healy, S., Tyrrell, M. (2011). Stress in Emergency Departments: Experiences of nurses and doctors. *Emergency Nurse*, 19(4), pp. 31–37.

Hooper, C., Craig, J., Janvrin, D.R., Wetsel, M.A., Reimels, E. (2010). Compassion satisfaction, burnout, and compassion fatigue among emergency nurses compared with nurses in other selected inpatient specialties. *Journal of Emergency Nursing*, 36(5), pp. 420–427.

Hussin, E.O.D., Wong, L.P., Chong, M.C., Subramanian, P. (2018). Factors associated with nurses' perceptions about quality of end-of-life care. *International Nursing Review*, 65(2), pp. 200–208.

Iserson, K.V. (2000). Notifying survivors about sudden, unexpected deaths. *The Western Journal of Medicine*, 173(4), pp. 261–265.

Jackson, V.A., Sullivan, A.M., Gadmer, N.M., Seltzer, D., Mitchell, A.M., Lakoma, M.D., Arnold, R.M., Block, S.D. (2005). "It was haunting…": Physicians' descriptions of emotionally powerful patient deaths. *Academic Medicine*, 80(7), pp. 648–656.

Keyes, K.M., Pratt, C., Galea, S., McLaughlin, K.A., Koenen, K.C., Shear, M.K. (2014). The burden of loss: Unexpected death of a loved one and psychiatric disorders across the life course in a national study. *Journal of American Psychiatry*, 171(8), pp. 864–871.

Kongsuwan, W., Matchim, Y., Nilmanat, K., Locsin, R.C., Tanioka, T., Yasuhara, Y. (2016). Lived experience of caring for dying patients in emergency room. *International Nursing Review*, 63(1), pp. 132–138.

Kutner, J.S., Kilbourn, K.M. (2009). Bereavement: Addressing challenges faced by advanced cancer patients, their caregivers and their physicians. *Primary Care*, 36(4), pp. 825–844.

Lai, X.B., Wong, F.K.Y., Ching, S.S.Y. (2018). The experience of caring for patients at the end-of-life stage in non-palliative care settings: A qualitative study. *BMC Palliative Care*, 17(1), p. 116.

Lin, Y., Long-Sutehall, T., Myall, M. (2021). Transferring home to die from critical care units: A scoping review of international practices. *Journal of Critical Care*, 65, pp. 205–215.

Linklater, G.T. (2010). Educational needs of foundation doctors caring for dying patients. *Journal of the Royal College of Physicians Edinburgh*, 40(1), pp. 13–18.

Loghmani, L., Borhani, F., Abbaszadeh, A. (2014). Factors affecting the nurse-patients' family communication in intensive care unit of Kerman: A qualitative study. *Journal of Caring Sciences*, 3(1), pp. 67–82.

Luder, H.U. (1993). Onset of human aging estimated from hazard functions associated with various causes of death. *Mechanisms of Ageing and Development*, 1993(67), pp. 247–259.

Mar Díaz-Cortés, M.D., Granero-Molina, J., Hernández-Padilla, J.M., Rodríguez, R.P., Casado, M.C., Fernández-Sola, C. (2018). Promoting dignified end-of-life care in the Emergency Department: A qualitative study. *International Emergency Nursing*, 37, pp. 23–28.

McDonald, S.M. (2012). Perception: A concept analysis. *International Journal of Nursing Knowledge*, 23(1), pp. 2–9.

McFarlane, A., Bryant, R. (2007). Post-traumatic stress disorder in occupational settings: Anticipating and managing the risk. *Occupational Medicine*, 57(6), pp. 404–410.

Meichenbaum, D. (1994). *A clinical handbook/practical therapist manual for assessing and treating adults with post-traumatic stress disorder*. Ontario: Institute Press.

Mierendorf, S.M., Gidvani, V. (2014). Palliative care in the Emergency Department. *The Permanente Journal*, 18(2), pp. 77–85.

Newson, R.S., Boelen, P.A., Hek, K., Hofman, A., Tiemeier, H. (2011). The prevalence and characteristics of complicated grief in older adults. *Journal of Affective Disorders*, 132(1–2), pp. 231–238.

NHS England (2020a). *Summary Hospital-level Mortality Indicator (SHMI) - Deaths associated with hospitalisation, England, September 2018-August 2019*. Available: https://digital.nhs.uk/data-and-information/publications/clinical-indicators/shmi/current (Accessed: 10 October 2024).

NHS England (2020b). *A&E attendances and emergency admissions 2019–20*. Available: https://www.england.nhs.uk/statistics/statistical-work-areas/ae-waiting-times-and-activity/ae-attendances-and-emergency-admissions-2019-20/ (Accessed: 10 October 2024).

NRS – National Records of Scotland (2018). *Vital events – Deaths*. Available: https://www.nrscotland.gov.uk/files//statistics/accidental-deaths/2018/accidental-deaths-18-main-points.pdf (Accessed: 12 October 2024).

Omoya, O., De Bellis, A., Breaden, K. (2022). Death, dying, and end-of-life care provision by doctors and nurses in the Emergency Department. *Journal of Hospice & Palliative Nursing*, 24(2), pp. 48–57.

ONS – Office for National Statistics (2015). *National Survey of Bereaved People (VOICES): England, 2015*. Available: https://www.ons.gov.uk/peoplepopulationandcommunity/healthandsocialcare/healthcaresystem/bulletins/nationalsurveyofbereavedpeoplevoices/england2015 (Accessed: 22 December 2024).

Park, H.J., Lee, Y.M., Won, M.H., Lim, S.J., Son, Y.J. (2020). Hospital nurses' perception of death and self-reported performance of end-of-life care: Mediating role of attitude towards end-of-life care. *Healthcare*, 8(2), p. 142.

Payne, S.A., Dean, S.J., Kalus, C. (1998). A comparative study of death anxiety in hospice and emergency nurses. *Journal of Advanced Nursing*, 28(4), pp. 700–706.

Peery, A.I. (2010). Caring and burnout in registered nurses: What's the connection? *International Journal for Human Caring*, 14(2), pp. 53–60.

Peters, L., Cant, R., Payne, S., O'Connor, M., McDermott, F., Hood, K., Morphet, J., Shimoinaba, K. (2013). Emergency and palliative care nurses' levels of anxiety about death and coping with death: A questionnaire survey. *Australasian Emergency Nursing Journal*, 16(4), pp. 152–159.

Pines, J.M., Hilton, J.A., Weber E.J. (2011). International perspectives on Emergency Department crowding. *Academic Emergency Medicine*, 18(12), pp. 1358–1370.

Pivodic, L., Pardon, K., Morin, L., Addington-Hall, J., Miccinesi, G., Cardenas-Turanzas, M. (2016). Place of death in the population dying from diseases indicative of palliative care need: A cross-national population-level study in 14 countries. *Journal of Epidemiology and Community Health*, 70(1), pp. 17–24.

Portnoy, D. (2011). Burnout and compassion fatigue: Watch for the signs. *Health Progress*, 92(4), pp. 46–50.

PRB – Population Reference Bureau (2019). *Fact sheet: Ageing in the United States.* Available: https://www.prb.org/aging-unitedstates-fact-sheet/ (Accessed: 12 February 2024).

Preston, S.H., Heuveline, P., Guillot, M. (2001). *Demography: Measuring and modelling population processes.* Oxford: Blackwell.

Public Health England (2018). *Statistical commentary: End of life care profiles, February 2018 update.* Available: https://www.gov.uk/government/publications/end-of-life-care-profiles-february-2018-update/statistical-commentary-end-of-life-care-profiles-february-2018-update (Accessed: 05 February 2024).

Redinbaugh, E.M., Sullivan, A.M., Block, S.D., Gadmer, N.M., Lakoma, M., Mitchell, A.M., Seltzer, D., Wolford, J., Arnold, R.M. (2003). Doctors' emotional reactions to recent death of a patient: Cross sectional study of hospital doctors. *British Medical Journal*, 327(7408), p. 185.

Riley, J.B. (2012). *Communication in nursing.* London: Mosby Elsevier.

Rosdahl, C.B., Kowalski, M.T. (2008). *Textbook of basic nursing* (Ninth Edition). Philadelphia, PA: Wolters Kluwer Health|Lippincott Williams & Wilkins.

Royal College of Emergency Medicine (2021). *RCEM acute insight series: Crowding and its consequences.* Available at: https://rcem.ac.uk/wp-content/uploads/2021/11/RCEM_Why_Emergency_Department_Crowding_Matters.pdf (Accessed: 03 December 2024).

Sadler, K., Abudari, G., Aljawi, D., Snelling, D. (2020). Deaths in the Emergency Department: An assessment of patient's end-of-life trajectory and quality of care. *Indian Journal of Palliative Care*, 26(3), pp. 352–357.

Salinari, G., De Santis, G. (2015). On the beginning of mortality acceleration. *Demography*, 2015(52), pp. 39–60.

Sanchez, B., Hirzel, A.H., Bingisser, R. (2013). State of emergency medicine in Switzerland: A national profile of Emergency Departments in 2006. *International Journal of Emergency Medicine*, 6(1), p. 23.

SBJ – Statistics Bureau of Japan (2019). *Statistical handbook of Japan 2019.* Available: https://www.stat.go.jp/english/data/handbook/c0117.html (Accessed: 12 February 2024).

Smulowitz, P.B., O'Malley, J., Yang, X., Landon, B.E. (2014). Increased use of the Emergency Department after health care reform in Massachusetts. *Annals of Emergency Medicine*, 64(2), pp. 107–115.

Strote, J., Schroeder, E., Lemos, J., Paganelli, R., Solberg, J., Range Hutson, H. (2011). Academic emergency physicians' experiences with patient death. *Academic Emergency Medicine*, 18(3), pp. 255–260.

UHS – University Hospital Southampton (2018). *Care at the end of life. Results of a survey of bereaved families*, July 2018. UHS.

Yingting, Z., Yash Pal, R., Wai, T., Wilson, S., Lee, A., Ong, M., Hwaa, T.L. (2018). Spiritual perspectives of emergency medicine doctors and nurses in caring for end-of-life patients: A mixed-method study. *International Emergency Nursing*, 37, pp. 13–22.

Zheng, R., Lee, S.F., Bloomer, M.J. (2018). How nurses cope with patient death: A systematic review and qualitative meta-synthesis. *Journal of Clinical Nursing*, 27(1–2), pp. 39–49.

Webb, L., Holland, K. (2011). *Nursing: Communication skills in practice*. London: Oxford University Press.

Whippen, D.A., Canellos, G.P. (1991). Burnout syndrome in the practice of oncology: Results of a random survey of 1,000 oncologists. *Journal of Clinical Oncology*, 9(10), pp. 1916–1920.

Chapter 3

Death and dying beyond the biological dimension

Values and norms are at the core of our identity and will define our actions, support us in decision-making, or help us navigate through complex situations. As these values are often rooted in our social and cultural backgrounds and are influenced by our spiritual and moral belief systems, discussing how death is perceived and interpreted among these dimensions will help us better understand healthcare professionals' death experiences. Understanding death beyond the biological dimension will start with exploring the social aspect of death, describing how social death builds certain activities around a patient in a hospital, how institutionalisation of death creates a detachment from social activities, healthcare professionals often treating progressively dying patients as being already dead. The cultural aspect of death will be discussed next, acknowledging how the Western concept of death is different from those in some other cultures, including cultures dominated by the views of different religions, how these cultures developed different ways to cope with death, creating often barriers and discomfort in healthcare professionals, when it comes to providing culturally sensitive end-of-life care. The spiritual aspect of death will explore how spirituality means more than simply religious beliefs, defining individual's search for purpose in life and meaning in death, how dying patients often experience an existential suffering, and how healthcare professionals can assist patients nearing death to alleviate death anxiety. The discussion in this chapter will conclude with presenting the ethical challenges healthcare professionals often face when caring for their dying patients, and how moral reasoning supports them to treat their patients with dignity and respect.

The social aspect of death

Birth and death are rites of passage experienced by every human, shared universally, and while describing death may seem simple, its meaning, and understanding as a concept are complex and vary, when considering the biological, social, cultural, spiritual, or moral aspects, making the examination of this behavioural phenomenon extremely complex. The complexity of concepts about death and dying originate in the challenge of defining what death means (Gire, 2014). Traditional biological approaches describe death as the absence of vital functions, such

DOI: 10.4324/9781032660912-3

as respiration or heartbeat, while modern life-sustaining technology has connected death to the cessation of brain functions (Neimeyer et al., 2003; Segen, 2006, Borgstrom, 2017).

Beyond the biological aspect, separation of the physical body from the invisible spirit, or the cessation of social activities and relationships of the dying, are two examples of additional dimensions that highlight a more holistic concept of death. As such, there may be no clear, identifiable point in time where a person can be considered to be dying (Davey, 2001).

In his seminal work, investigating the social aspect of death and dying in a hospital setting, the American sociologist, David Sudnow claims that dying is not a straightforward term, as we are all in the process of dying from the moment of birth (Sudnow, 1967). Even death as a medical event is subject to controversy among physicians, as some will claim that represents the moment of cessation of cellular activity, while others relate that to properties of cellular multiplication. The social context of dying is given by links to a variety of thoughts, concerns, emotions, and activities, which relates to that person's location along the temporal dimension of social structures. According to Sudnow, 'dying' builds a frame of social activities around the patient, and this includes the hospital environment too. These social activities could include allowing visitors at any time, termination of certain medical treatments, start of rites and final prayers in case of a religious person, or taking the patient into register for a possible autopsy, while the patient is still alive (Sudnow, 1967).

One of the first observations made by Sudnow was related to the institutionalisation of death. The process of converting 'dealing with death' into a norm or convention was depicted by stocking equipment, such as morgue trays, death sheets, or relevant documentation bundles on a regular basis on wards, suggesting that death is regarded as a recurrent daily happening. Another aspect was the way staff was referring to death during shift handovers, staff meetings, or ordinary conversations, talking about deceased patients as a statistical indicator. Although staff regarded 'common death' as an ordinary event, there were always dramatic cases, such as a certain unexpected death, the death of a child or a celebrity, which served as subject to ward gossip, being remembered for a longer period. Another initial observation made by the author was in relation to the general attitude, especially observed within nursing and medical students, about witnessing death as being perceived as a sign of maturity. Once somebody starts witnessing death on a regular basis, soon will reach a point, when will 'stop counting'. Sudnow observed, following several interviews, that the highest number of deaths, anyone could remember before 'losing count', was 8, death often being discussed in reference with a similar event in the past (Sudnow, 1967).

Sudnow suggests that from the moment of 'social death' hospital staff will treat the patient as someone who is 'already dead'. Sudnow also highlights how moral presumptions can influence clinical decision-making. A patient who is drunk causing a car accident or someone who tried committing suicide was less likely to receive the same effort for revival, in case of a trauma, compared to a child or a young, otherwise healthy adult, during the time his observations were made, in

America of the 1960s (Sudnow, 1967). Timmermans (1998) revisited Sudnow's work, to investigate whether the radical changes in healthcare systems, such as the rationalisation of medical practices or the wider focus on patient autonomy, made social rationing as described by Sudnow (1967) irrelevant. Timmermans argued that these changes, on the contrary, have contributed to the development of further inequalities, surrounding death and dying. Discussing resuscitation efforts, he suggests that the Emergency Department (ED) staff often needs to balance clinical knowledge, boundaries of the law and professional ethics to allow some to live and others to die a dignified death, while much often resuscitation practice "becomes an attempt to avoid a lawsuit as an endeavour to save lives".

As resuscitation became a repetitive and frequent practice in the ED, developing into an "empty ritual", Timmermans (1998) noted that staff started displaying detachment from their patients, and only when they regained personhood, was that staff intended to "aggressively try to revive them". Interested in the social construction of death, Seale (1998) argues that social life involves turning towards life and away from the inevitability of death. According to Seale (1998), social activities are able to provide security and meaning to an existence threatened by the knowledge of mortality. From a sociological perspective, Seale views death as posing a challenge on two levels, in threatening stability of social structures and in the maintenance of individual meanings. 'Hiding away' represents an attitude of 'death denial' in the modern societies, resulting from the observation that people who biologically die have usually experienced a social death preceding this. This social death is largely supported by the institutionalisation of death, including disengagement from active social participation of the elderly, and the management or physical segregation of those dying in the healthcare system. This attitude of 'death denial' is often explained by becoming free to concentrate on the issues of the living, without considering the needs of the dead (Seale, 1998).

The cultural aspect of death

The importance of examining cultural variations in attitudes towards death and dying is related to the significance of how people act in life and how they approach death, allowing healthcare professionals to have a more in-depth understanding about individual concepts of death, experiences of grief, or burial rituals, knowledge that can become integral part of their patient care. Individual experiences of death and dying, loss and behaviours of grieving, after the death of a loved one, and the way these feelings are expressed may differ across cultures (Jensen, 2015). A culture represents a mix of values, beliefs, traditions, behaviours, and rituals shared among members of the same cultural group (Cacciatore and DeFrain, 2015). Culture specific traditions surrounding death provide a set of directions that help structure people's roles during this time of death (Jensen, 2015). As described earlier in this chapter, defining a unified concept of death is almost impossible. The largely Western concept of death, including the medical definition of this concept, is rooted in eight criteria, which incorporates the lack of spontaneous respiration or response to various stimuli, lack of motor reflexes, and a flat electroencephalogram (EEG)

Table 3.1 The eight criteria to determine whole-brain death

No.	*Criteria to determine whole-brain death*
1	**No spontaneous movement** in response to any stimuli
2	**No spontaneous respiration** for at least one hour
3	**Total lack of responsiveness** to even the most painful stimuli
4	**No eye movements**, blinking, or pupil responses
5	**No postural activity**, swallowing, yawning, or vocalising
6	**No motor reflexes**
7	**A flat electroencephalogram** (EEG) for at least ten minutes
8	**No change in any of these criteria** when tested again 24 hours later

for at least ten minutes, all of which needs to be met before death is confirmed. All eight criteria commonly used in Western medicine to determine whole-brain death are listed in Table 3.1.

On the contrary, in some South Pacific cultures, life is seen as departing the body when someone is ill or asleep, as such a person is 'dying several times' prior to their final death (Gire, 2014). In cultures where faith and religion are important aspects of everyday life, societies in which most people share the same religion, these beliefs significantly shape the culture (Lobar et al., 2006). Components of the culture shape the ways of defining, interpreting, and understanding the meaning and purpose of life and what happens after death, which could serve as an indication to healthcare professionals how people in those cultures approach or what their attitude is about death (Lobar et al., 2006). Hinduism, for example, sees life as a cycle, where death is only an opportunity to be reborn with a new identity, even multiple times. In contrast, in Christianity and Islam, death occurs only once, and while a person ceases to exist in their physical body, they continue to exist in a spiritual realm. According to some segments of Buddhism and some Native American tribes, the dead and living co-exist, the dead often impacting the life of those living (Gire, 2014). These elements specific to a culture include its own rituals that influence the expression of mourning and grief, which are meant to offer a sense of stability and security, when carried out (Jensen, 2015). While death can create a sense of chaos and confusion, because of the experienced loss, traditions and rituals are meant to provide a sense of routine and steadiness. Death is part of a natural life cycle; as such, all cultures have developed ways to cope with the experience of death, while obstructing or interfering with these practices can disturb people's ability to cope, during this complex process (Cacciatore and DeFrain, 2015). Grief responses within a culture vary from person to person, as often people, to meet their unique needs, will adapt the beliefs and values of their culture within the current circumstances (Lobar et al., 2006).

In some cultures, relatives wear black or white as a sign of mourning, often for a prolonged period of time, while in other cultures, often for a lifetime. Some cultures require close relatives to shave their heads or marry the spouse of the deceased. Yet, in other cultures, an alternative expression of mourning, a celebration of the life of the deceased is expressed through dancing, eating, and drinking. Despite cultural rituals surrounding death, emotional reactions and human reactions to the experience of death, for example, through crying or anger are considered universal (Gire, 2014). This experience is often shared in a Western society, which is made up of people from various cultural backgrounds, when a person's experience of grief may be at odds with the widely accepted cultural norms. For example, crying in public might feel uncomfortable for some, while others may have a level of despair that, within the given cultural norms, might feel out of step (Lobar et al., 2006).

Healthcare professionals are not expected to know the mourning ceremonies and traditions of every culture; however, a basic understanding of how different cultures respond to death is important, as it could shape their experience and attribute meaning to death (Cacciatore and DeFrain, 2015). Acculturation is undoubtably paramount for healthcare professionals in determining the beliefs and values of a family, coping, and mourning the death of a loved one, so that both the preparation for death and post-death arrangements meet their individual needs (Robben, 2017). In general, beliefs about the meaning of death help people make sense of it, and cope with the unknown. For example, people who believe in life after death may find death more bearable, or family members often could be comforted by the belief that their loved one is watching over them (Cacciatore and DeFrain, 2015). Healthcare professionals could experience a sense of discomfort when it comes to providing culturally sensitive end-of-life or bereavement care, especially if language and cultural barriers add to the challenges of remaining both professionally appropriate and compassionate (Swihart et al., 2021). While families experiencing a loss could need guidance and compassion from healthcare professionals, often the realities of a busy environment such as the ED could cause people to simply fail in the moment, to express sufficient warmth and sensitivity. In our Westernised societies, a logical linear thinking is natural when critical decisions must be made, yet for many people from different cultures, a direct approach straight after death, for example, related to organ donation, may appear as inhumane and harsh (Swihart et al., 2021).

The spiritual aspect of death

Spirituality is a broad concept, looking above the physical aspect of human life and refers to how individuals search for meaning and purpose in life, and connectedness to the self, others, and the environment (Beauregard and O'Leary, 2009). Spirituality often establishes its importance when someone is experiencing physical illness, emotional stress, or death, and could incorporate elements of religious beliefs (Pulchaski et al., 2009). The importance of spirituality reflects in finding a connection to something greater than ourselves, resulting in a positive state of mind and emotions, such as gratitude, peace, or acceptance, crucial when someone is experiencing death (Beauregard and O'Leary, 2009). However, most hospital environments, having an emphasis to cure patients, tend to focus on the physical aspects of illness, while dying patients are confronted with complex challenges, including their spiritual integrity and wellbeing (Costello, 2006; Balboni et al., 2010).

Dying patients often experience a spiritual and existential suffering, which may have a profound impact on the wellbeing of family members, often devastating because it prompts their awareness of loss. This suffering can be described as an anguish that may include concerns related to hopelessness, remorse, meaninglessness, a disruption of personal identity, or a general experience of 'death anxiety' in patients and may trigger grief, depression, and anxiety in family members (Bruce et al., 2011). Alleviating dying patients' death anxiety and distress is possible through spiritual care, which may include religious and other existential aspects (Kisvetrová et al., 2013). 'Death anxiety' is a term difficult to define, as it can include the fear of death of oneself or others, having different meanings when is examined at private or public levels. Due to its complexity, death anxiety has also a cultural aspect, some cultures managing the idea of someone dying relatively well, being defined as 'death affirming cultures', while other cultures are referred to as 'death-defying cultures', being described by an avoidant attitude towards death. Western societies, incorporating more material traditions, in general could be described as 'death-defying', as talking about death largely remains an uncomfortable subject, while Eastern cultural beliefs, holding often strong spiritual characteristics, generally view death as a mere transition, accepting death as part of life (Gire, 2014). Creating a compassionate and caring environment that brings hope and help patients to deal with the reality of death will involve interventions conveying empathy, active listening, assisting patients to accept their own feelings about dying, being present and showing respect, while advocating for patient dignity (Tanyi, 2006).

Healthcare professionals often experience that the spiritual and existential suffering of their dying patients emerge as a complex embodiment of various pains, including the physical, mental, emotional, relational, or spiritual aspect (Norberg et al., 2001). Healthcare professionals can assist patients nearing death to alleviate anxiety and achieve reconciliation with themselves, the family, or with God, resolve family conflicts, settle unfinished affairs, or eliminate worries, peacefulness in dying patients often being the result of a feeling of 'completion' and 'closure' (Gijsberts et al., 2019). Nurses sometimes have mixed feelings about providing spiritual care, due to lack of time, the constant risk of being interrupted, and the insufficient available resources, although most of them would agree that this aspect of care being very important (Steinhauser et al., 2000).

Hesitation to provide support with the spiritual or existential needs of their patients often roots in relating this care purely to religion or religious beliefs. Sometimes nurses use this as an excuse to avoid the challenge of talking with patients about their spiritual concerns, especially if they don't consider themselves to be religious, or feel that believes and faith are very personal matters (Tornøe et al., 2015). The qualities allowing nurses to provide spiritual care are rooted in their life experience, professional experience working with dying patients and their families, advanced communication skills and their perception of reality, that develops from personal spirituality. These qualities of spiritual care enable healthcare professionals to identify and address spiritual needs of their patients, and encourages patients to disclose and co-process these spiritual needs (Batstone et al., 2020). Spiritual and existential suffering sometimes will emerge spontaneously, such as during personal care or any other time when nurses are able to focus and take time to actively listen. Nurses' ability to concentrate on the arising moments, when patients wanted and needed to express their thoughts and feelings, is seen as an essential nursing skill that helps patients to alleviate their spiritual and existential suffering, which can be understood as an alienation or a threat against a person's connectedness and their sense of identity and integrity (Tornøe et al., 2015; Norberg et al., 2001).

Ethical and moral challenges

Understanding the role of individual moral values and how they are shaped by larger structures of ethical constructs, existing in a profession, an institution or society, will offer a better insight into how individual experiences of death in the ED could be influenced by these values. Morality incorporates personal values and the rules of behaviour regulating social intercourse, having at the centre interpersonal relationships, and striving to treat other human beings with dignity and respect, while promoting welfare, creativity and meaning (Doris, 2010). Individual moral values are action-oriented beliefs, about truth, beauty, and worth, giving direction and purpose to the individual (Carvalho et al., 2011). Moral values are more than an external structure, they are bonded in our identity and understanding of who we are as a person; as such, it is not something we lightly step in and out of. Without a moral order, the individual finds it difficult to interpret and make sense of the surrounding reality. It is argued that personal values are not static, and they form a hierarchy, prioritising some values before others, becoming instruments in making decisions (Joas, 2000; Lapsley, 2009). The major differences between values and norms are listed in Table 3.2.

In the process of developing a moral self in which the individual navigates and internalises the norms, meanings, and language with which interprets the world, needs to define communities that will constitute a framework for this process,

Table 3.2 The key differences between values and norms

Feature	*Values*	*Norms*
Nature	*Abstract*: Not tied to specific actions or situations	*Concrete*: Specific to actions and contexts
Function	*Guiding principles*: Influence behaviour and decision-making	*Guiding principles*: Tell people how to act in given situations
Enforcement	*Internal* (conscience, identity)	*External* (social pressure)
Flexibility	More stable over time	More adaptable to context

establishing shared values within those communities (Solbrekke and Jensen, 2006). Moral order represents a value system that differentiates right, good, and desirable from bad, improper, and immoral. This moral order develops over a lifetime and originates from a variety of sources, being influenced by a series of geographical, anthropological, sociological, psychological, and theological factors (Doris, 2010). Moral reasoning in healthcare professionals is a mental process which is applied to set in motion a decision-making effort, making a distinction between 'right' and 'wrong' in any moral dilemma. While values, in general, are interpreted as motivational preferences or dispositions, moral values for healthcare professionals represent those preferences that are aligned with a moral reasoning (Austin, 2007). Individual moral values are defined by commitments to, and identification with the moral orders of the communities to which the individual belongs. In this sense, healthcare professionals' personal values are influenced by the moral order of the wider society, the medical or nursing profession's norms, the healthcare institution, and the clinical ward where they work.

Personal morality of a healthcare professional will develop through engagement and exchange with others in the communities in which they participate (Carvalho et al., 2011).

A literature review of nursing ethical values and definitions, reflecting on observations from studies originating in 12 countries, has found that the ten most commonly shared values in nursing are: human dignity, altruism, social justice, autonomy in decision-making, precision and accuracy in caring, responsibility, human relationship, individual and professional competency, sympathy, and trust (Shahriari et al., 2013). A hierarchy of values represents a structure, where one value is at the top of the priorities while others have less importance. In the healthcare professions, the priority of certain values will never change, such as the standard of treating people as individuals, which require healthcare professionals not to discriminate in any form, against those in their care (Pullman, 2004). Another value that may also never change is the conscientious objection, which relates to issues contrary to a nurse's moral beliefs and values, such as sanctity of life, on which nobody should be expected to compromise (Lloyd and Cooley, 2014). While some values can represent an individual's bedrock value that will never change, whatever the circumstances, other values could be more flexible and adaptable. A clarification and self-assessment of our own values can help us understand why a particular person (e.g., a healthcare professional or a patient), or circumstances affect us in a certain way. Nurses who fail to examine and articulate their personal values may not be fully effective in their provision of care for their patients (Carvalho et al., 2011). While there is an expectation towards nurses to be 'non-judgemental', personal values will create a framework upon which they judge others. Yet, these judgements must not be allowed to influence a nurse's professional manner (Kaldjian, 2013).

Personal values and moral standpoints taken will also define the outcome of dealing with problems that arise in healthcare, many of them being related to honesty, doing good, valuing someone's worth, or being fair in a situation (Moyo et al., 2016). Healthcare professionals are expected to provide anti-discriminatory patient care, thus issues such as accountability, responsibility, and negligence during this process will have to be explored in the context of professional and personal values (NMC, 2015). Similarly to nurses, doctors practise an ethically driven profession, as their purpose is to improve the health of their patients. They are often faced by a variety of ethical and moral decision-making situations, which should be guided by principles, such as focusing on the outcomes or consequences of these decisions, while giving priority to the inner values of the decision-maker. Principles that are expected doctors to be engaged with, when confronting moral dilemmas in medical practice include self-determination, competence, confidentiality, honesty, benefit-seeking, and fairness. An example of self-determination is the ability to refuse any proposed medical intervention, even where the decision may result in death, justified by the anticipated benefits exceeding the potential harms (Ashcroft et al., 2007). A study conducted among doctors of all specialities found that 62% of them agreed that receiving futile and invasive investigations or treatments for patients near death is very common, mainly because preserving and lengthening life is the default medical approach (Visser, 2012). A moral and ethical dilemma often encountered by doctors is when they do not provide treatments or medical interventions, which are unlikely to benefit a patient at the end of their life, guided by the intention to preserve their dignity (Marck et al., 2014).

Human dignity, as an aspect of morality, can be explained and defined alongside numerous competing concepts, taking their meaning from a political, cosmological, religious, or anthropological aspect. The German philosopher Immanuel Kant (1785) argues that a person during their life, including the end of it, must feel that it lived a dignified life. In his view, the autonomy of the individual represents the central element of dignity, something to which every human being has a right. Despite the many differences in interpretation, human dignity in general relates to the ideas of sanctity, autonomy, personhood, flourishing, and self-respect of the individual. Having dignity should be recognised and maintained in every human being, reflecting the individual's choices, ideals, values, and lifestyles (Formosa, 2014). Dignity is also a social construction that regulates our relationship with others, defined by attributes such as respect, empowerment, autonomy, and communication, alongside feeling comfortable with oneself and having control over one's decisions, choices, and surroundings (Haugen, 2010). Dignity of a human being is also extended to the process of dying. Dying with dignity represents a priority for patients, their families, and the care providers, also being recognised as an essential objective for palliative and end-of-life care, although it might be sometimes unintentionally overlooked (Griffin-Heslin, 2005). Chochinov's (2002) model for preserving dignity of a patient has identified several characteristics that can influence the patient's sense of dignity. The model identifies three major areas that define the subject of dignity in end-of-life care, namely, the patient's ability to satisfy themselves their own needs, within the context of the symptoms suffered; prerequisites and actions to preserve patient dignity; and the social context that influence the patient's dignity.

The most important focus in the ED context is to provide urgent life-saving medical treatment in the hope of minimising morbidity, prevent death, and improve patient's overall clinical condition and wellbeing. While this ethos remains the primary goal for the ED, end-of-life care is recognised as a core task for ED healthcare professionals, with dignity as a pivotal element of this care (Quest, et al., 2011). Yet, ED clinicians repeatedly reported dignity of the patient being in danger, due to a conflict arising from the life-saving ethos characteristic to ED and providing end-of-life care in the same environment (Grudzen et al., 2012a, b). This fast-paced environment can constantly create situations surrounding death and dying, that could be the source of ethical and moral challenges. These may arise from clinical judgements that contradict family wishes, clinical interventions prioritised over holistic care, different interpretations of 'quality of life', or ED resources being focused on life-saving procedures, rather than palliation. Ethical and moral dilemmas are frequently raised in emergency situations, especially when the clinical rationale of a case presentation, from the healthcare professional perspective, contradicts the wishes of the patient, or their close family. A case study of an end-of-life patient, reported by an emergency doctor in a Singapore hospital, is a prime example of the moral complexity of a clinical decision, taking into consideration the clinical realities, the perceived wishes of the patient, and the conflicting demands of the closest family members (Siddiqui, 2016).

The patient in his late 60s presented with shortness of breath and fever at the ED, having a history of nasopharyngeal carcinoma. The patient also had an Advanced Medical Directive (AMD), a legal document that informs a doctor, in the event of becoming terminally ill and unconscious, that life-sustaining treatment should not be used to prolong life (similar to the DNACPR – Do Not Attempt Cardiopulmonary Resuscitation – document used in the UK). The patient's AMD clearly stated that in case of dying from cancer, he does not wish to have invasive or mechanical ventilation. A moral conflict arose as the patient's family demanded the medical team to do everything in their power to save his life, against the patient's documented wishes. Family wishes were granted, and after two days spent in intensive care, with the family at his bedside and once the irreversibility was established, the treatment was discontinued, and the patient died. The family members were reported being at peace with the decision, offering everyone the possibility to say goodbye and have their closure. The study acknowledges that in similar situations the "line between right and wrong is often blurred" in the ED. On one side, there were the clinical risks associated with the intervention and the documented wishes of the patient against being intubated. On the other side, the distress of the family, not being ready to 'let go' of their son, husband, and father. The case study raises the dilemma that the unconscious patient potentially would have agreed with the treatment if he would have known, that he spares his family from unnecessary social harm and emotional pain. The case study further suggests that principles of autonomy and non-maleficence should be applied not only to the patient, but also as relational, contextual principles, to the extended family, taking into consideration, not only the physical aspect, but also other elements of individual wellbeing (Siddiqui, 2016).

Similar conflicts between staff and family members are often seen by healthcare professionals working in the ED as inevitable, and that communication and conflict resolution skills are required to resolve such situations. Conflicts are often resolved by allowing patients and their family to have all their questions answered and clarified or by offering them the experience and the feeling of being heard. Transferring a patient from the ED to intensive care for a slow removal of invasive treatment instead of a sudden and determinant decision to stop all treatment in the ED could be also seen as a measure of allowing the family to accept the inevitable death of their loved one (Omoya et al., 2022). Ethical dilemmas surrounding the course of actions related to an end-of-life patient in the ED occur more often when the wishes of the patient and their family are unknown. The dilemma is often fuelled by a conflict with the doctors, who consider only medical treatment as a course of actions, while nurses may try to act as advocates on behalf of the patient. Nurses often argue that they experience "discomfort with feelings of distress, suffering, anger and helplessness in these situations" (Jimenez-Herrera and Axelsson, 2015). Similar ethical controversies are regularly experienced when the option of treatments offered to patients nearing death in the ED, considered futile by some clinicians, contradicts the principles of 'quality life' and 'quality death' (Omoya et al., 2022). The decision to consider a treatment futile is not always 'black and white' and should be based not only on clinical considerations, but weighed individually, looking into the ethical aspect of each case. For example, an invasive treatment could prove futile for an 80-year-old, living a 'low quality' life, the same treatment prolonging the life of a 34 years old with a month, to see her daughter's first birthday, would fall under a different moral category. Quality of life or death should also be defined by the dying patient and not accounted as what a healthcare professional working in the ED would imagine as being for that individual patient (Omoya et al., 2022).

When a patient has a cardiac arrest, the first decision to be made is to whether to start resuscitation, and if resuscitation is started, what is the likelihood that resuscitation will bring the patient back to a 'good quality life' or not. While the decision taken must be immediate, the ethical dilemma will persist up until the outcome and even after. The same dilemma within the context of healthcare professionals working in the ED, being trained to save lives, raises the question of defending life at all costs, potentially leading to not 'allowing' people to die and denying their right to do so in a dignified way (Jimenez-Herrera and Axelsson, 2015). These dilemmas are permanently influenced by the healthcare professionals' cultural and religious views and beliefs about death and dying, especially when those are shared with the dying patient and their family. As reported by one of the nurses in an Australian study: "I think those situations were easier maybe because I felt like they (the dying patient and families) were behaving the way I would behave" (Omoya et al., 2022).

Lack of emergency nurse's autonomy to exercise their professional role and of the patients in decision-making about their course of treatment is a further source of ethical and moral challenges. These dilemmas are mostly evident when doctors and nurses in the ED do not share the same view, doctors being mainly concerned with the biomedical aspect of a dying patient, while nurses' approach is more holistic (Jimenez-Herrera and Axelsson, 2015). On the other hand, both ED nurses and doctors consider the role of nurses carrying more responsibilities, doctors believing that it is very intensive from a nursing point of view to keep the end-of-life patients comfortable, while communicating with kindness. ED doctors who identified themselves as being 'an extension of the nurse's role' when it comes to end-of-life care, contradicted nurses, who often felt that once the end-of-life status was determined in the ED, care was relinquished to them by doctors. Other nurses felt that at this point doctors can't offer more to patients, while nurses will offer emotional support as part of their care (Omoya et al., 2022). Similarly to nurses, junior doctors often express their moral concerns over expectation by their more senior colleagues to move on from the care of the dying patients, once they were confirmed of being admitted to a ward, despite being physically still in the ED. As a result, the dying patient is given a lower care priority in the ED and is neglected by medical staff, resources being redirected to life-saving procedures and acute emergencies, making doctors feel uncomfortable about not going back to look after their dying patient. Nurses often also reflect that when a patient presented with the possibility of dying, clinical care came first, while emotional support for the end-of-life patient only occurred later, as this was "the only way to do the job" (Omoya et al., 2022).

Reference list

Ashcroft, R., Dawson, A., Draper, H., McMillan J. (2007). *Principles of health care ethics.* Chichester: John Wiley and Sons.

Austin, W. (2007). The ethics of everyday practice: Healthcare environments as moral communities. *Advances in Nursing Science*, 30(1), pp. 81–88.

Balboni, T.A., Paulk, M.E., Balboni, M.J., Phelps, A.C., Loggers, E.T., Wright, A.A. (2010). Provision of spiritual care to patients with advanced cancer: Associations with medical care and quality of life near death. *Journal of Clinical Oncology*, 28(3), pp. 445–452.

Batstone, E., Bailey, C., Hallett, N. (2020). Spiritual care provision to end-of-life patients: A systematic literature review. *Journal of Clinical Nursing*, 29(19–20), pp. 3609–3624.

Beauregard, M., O'Leary, D. (2009). *The spiritual brain.* New York: Harper Collins.

Borgstrom, E. (2017). Social death. *QJM: An International Journal of Medicine*, 110(1), pp. 5–7.

Bruce, A., Schreiber, R., Petrovskaya, O., Boston, P. (2011). Longing for ground in a ground (less) world: A qualitative inquiry of existential suffering. *BMC Nursing*, 10(1), p. 2.

Cacciatore, J., DeFrain, J. (2015). *The world of bereavement. Cultural perspectives on death in families.* New York: Springer.

Carvalho, S., Reeves, M., Orford, J. (2011). *Fundamental aspects of legal, ethical and professional issues in nursing* (Second Edition). Salisbury: Quay Books.

Chochinov, H.M. (2002). Dignity-conserving care – A new model for palliative care. *JAMA – Journal of American Medical Association*, 287(17), pp. 2253–2260.

Costello, J. (2006). Dying well: Nurses' experiences of 'good and bad' deaths in hospital. *Journal of Advanced Nursing*, 54(5), pp. 594–601.

Davey, B. (2001). Do-not-resuscitate decisions: Too many, too few, too late? *Mortality*, 6(3), pp. 247–264.

Doris, J.M. (2010). *The moral psychology handbook.* Oxford: Oxford University Press.
Formosa, P. (2014). Dignity and respect: How to apply Kant's formula of humanity. *The Philosophical Forum*, 45(1), pp. 49–68.
Gijsberts, M.H.E., Liefbroer, A.I., Otten, R., Olsman, E. (2019). Spiritual care in palliative care: A systematic review of the recent European literature. *Medical Sciences*, 7(2), p. 25.
Gire, J. (2014). How death imitates life: Cultural influences on conceptions of death and dying. *Online Readings in Psychology and Culture*, 6(2). https://doi.org/10.9707/2307-0919.1120
Griffin-Heslin, V.L. (2005). An analysis of the concept dignity. *Accident and Emergency Nursing*, 13(4), pp. 251–257.
Grudzen, C.R., Lynne, D.R., Hannah, M.M., Brandon, K., Joanna, M.O., Morrison, R.S. (2012a). Hospital administrators' views on barriers and opportunities to delivering palliative care in the Emergency Department. *Annals of Emergency Medicine*, 61(6), pp. 654–660.
Grudzen, C.R., Richardson, L.D., Susan, S.H., Joanna, M.O., Christine, W., Morrison, R.S. (2012b). Does palliative care have a future in the Emergency Department? Discussions with attending emergency physicians. *Journal of Pain Symptom Management*, 43(1), pp. 1–9.
Haugen, H.M. (2010). Inclusive and relevant language: The use of the concepts of autonomy, dignity and vulnerability in different contexts. *Medicine, Healthcare and Philosophy*, 13(3), pp. 203–213.
Jensen, L.A. (2015). *The Oxford handbook of human development and culture. An interdisciplinary perspective.* Oxford: The Oxford Press.
Jimenez-Herrera, M.F., Axelsson, Ć. (2015). Some ethical conflicts in emergency care. *Nursing Ethics*, 22(5), pp. 548–560.
Joas, H. (2000). *The genesis of values.* Chicago, IL: University of Chicago Press.
Kaldjian, L.C. (2013). Communicating moral reasoning in medicine as an expression of respect for patients and integrity among professionals. *Communication Medicine*, 10(2), pp. 177–183.
Kant, I. (1785). *Groundwork of the metaphysics of morals.* Translated and edited by M. Gregor, first published in 1998. Cambridge: Cambridge University Press.
Kisvetrová, H., Klugar, M., Kabelka, L. (2013). Spiritual support interventions in nursing care for patients suffering death anxiety in the final phase of life. *International Journal of Palliative Nursing*, 19(12), p. 599.
Lapsley, D.K. (2009). *Personality, identity and character. Exploration in moral psychology.* Cambridge: Cambridge University Press.
Lloyd, S., Cooley, D.R. (2014). *The ethics of death: Religious and philosophical perspectives in dialogue.* Washington, DC: Fortress Press.
Lobar, S.L., Youngblut, J.M., Brooten, D. (2006). Cross-cultural beliefs, ceremonies, and rituals surrounding death of a loved one. *Paediatric Nursing*, 32(1), pp. 44–50.
Marck, C.H., Weil, J., Lane, H., Weiland, T.J., Philip, J., Boughey, M., Jelinek, G.A. (2014). Care of the dying cancer patient in the Emergency Department: Findings from a national survey of Australian Emergency Department clinicians. *Internal Medicine Journal*, 44(4), pp. 362–368.
Moyo, M., Goodyear-Smith, F.A., Weller, J., Robb, G., Shulruf, B. (2016). Healthcare practitioners' personal and professional values. *Advances in Health Sciences Education*, 21(2), pp. 257–286.
Neimeyer, R.A., Moser, R.P., Winkowski, J. (2003). Assessing attitudes toward dying and death: Psychometric considerations. *Omega: Journal of Death and Dying*, 47(1), pp. 45–76.

NMC: Nursing and Midwifery Council (2015). *The code. Standards of conduct, performance and ethics for nurses and midwives.* Available at: https://www.nmc-uk.org/Documents/Standards/nmcTheCodeStandardsofConductPerformanceAndEthicsForNursesAndMidwives_LargePrintVersion.PDF (Accessed: 22 February 2024).

Norberg, A., Bergsten, M., Lundman, B. (2001). A model of consolation. *Nursing Ethics*, 8(6), pp. 544–553.

Omoya, O., De Bellis, A., Breaden, K. (2022). Death, dying, and end-of-life care provision by doctors and nurses in the Emergency Department. *Journal of Hospice & Palliative Nursing*, 24(2), pp. 48–57.

Pulchaski, C.M., Ferrell, B., Virani, R., Otis-Green, S. (2009). Improving the quality of spiritual care as a dimension of palliative care: The report of the consensus conference. *Journal of Palliative Medicine*, 12(10), pp. 886–904.

Pullman, D. (2004). Death, dignity, and moral nonsense. *Journal of Palliative Care*, 20(3), pp. 171–178.

Quest, T.E., Asplin, B.R., Cairns, C.B., Hwang, U., Pines, J.M. (2011). Research priorities for palliative and end-of-life care in the emergency setting. *Academic Emergency Medicine*, 18(6), pp. 70–76.

Robben, A.C. (2017). *Death, mourning and burial. A cross-cultural reader* (Second Edition). London: Wiley Blackwell.

Seale, C. (1998). *Constructing death. Sociology of dying and bereavement.* Cambridge: Cambridge University Press.

Segen, J.C. (2006). *Concise dictionary of modern medicine.* New York:The McGraw-Hill Companies.

Shahriari, M., Mohammadi, E., Abbaszadeh, A., Bahrami, M. (2013). Nursing ethical values and definitions: A literature review. *Iranian Journal of Nursing and Midwifery Research*, 18(1), pp. 1–8.

Siddiqui, S. (2016). A physician's moral dilemma in the Emergency Department: Going against a patient's perceived wishes. *The Journal of Emergency Medicine*, 51(6), pp. 748–749.

Solbrekke, T.D., Jensen, K. (2006). Learning the moral order of professions; the contrasting approaches of nursing and clinical psychology. *Learning in Health and Social Care*, 5(4), pp. 181–193.

Steinhauser, K.E., Christakis, N.A., Clipp, E.C., McNeilly, M., McIntyre, L., Tulsky, J.A. (2000). Factors considered important at the end of life by patients, family, physicians, and other care providers. *The Journal of the American Medical Association*, 284(19), pp. 2476–2482.

Sudnow, D. (1967). *Passing on.* Hoboken, NJ: Prentice-Hall.

Swihart, D.L., Yarrarapu, S., Martin, R.L. (2021). *Cultural religious competence in clinical practice.* Treasure Island, FL: StatPearls Publishing.

Tanyi, R.A. (2006). Spirituality and family nursing: Spiritual assessment and interventions for families. *Journal of Advanced Nursing*, 53(3), pp. 287–294.

Timmermans, S. (1998). Social death as self-fulfilling prophecy: David Sudnow's passing on revisited. *The Sociological Quarterly*, 39(3), pp. 453–472.

Tornøe, K.A., Danbolt, L.J., Kvigne, K., Sørlie, V. (2015). The challenge of consolation: Nurses' experiences with spiritual and existential care for the dying - A phenomenological hermeneutical study. *BMC Nursing*, 14, p. 62.

Visser, J. (2012). The doctor is in treatment mode. *Medical Contact*, 67, pp. 1326–1329.

Chapter 4

The complex process of bereavement

The subject of death in the Western societies in the first half of the 20th century was largely an uncomfortable topic, and something not to be discussed. Elisabeth Kübler-Ross was a Swiss-American psychiatrist, a pioneer in near-death studies, and author of the internationally best-selling book, *On Death and Dying* (1969), observed that people at the end of their life rarely had the opportunity to share their anxiety, feelings, fears, or emotions, sometimes even with the closest members of the family. Kübler-Ross suggests that instead of avoiding, isolating, or ignoring the dying or the bereaved, it is important to allow them to speak honestly and openly about their situation, understanding the individual stages of grief they are personally going through (Kübler-Ross, 1969; Morris, 2011; Kaplow et al., 2010).

Sudden death represents a form of death that is unexpected in its nature or timing, and the term can be applied when someone that is seemingly fit and well dies unexpectedly, but also includes people on a palliative trajectory, who die sooner than expected (Howarth, 2007). Bereavement, caused by a death that is unexpected, can be a stressful life experience, associated with the development of psychiatric disorders (Newson et al., 2011). The period of bereavement following a death can be complicated by circumstances such as unexpected or violent death, suicide, traumatic death, being unprepared for death, or the lack of a support system (Schoenberger et al., 2013).

While uncomplicated grief incorporates multiple responses, including emotional, cognitive, physical, and behavioural, as common reactions after a loss, the COVID-19 pandemic has rapidly changed the experiences of grief (Wallace et al., 2020). People's loss of a loved one during the pandemic may be complicated by a loss of financial security, loss of social and physical connections, loss of mental and physical health, and loss of autonomy, because of lockdown measures (Torrens-Burton et al., 2022). In the context of higher mortality rates during the pandemic, experiences of death may have been more frequent, potentially increasing exposure to, and impact of deaths in clinical settings (Das et al., 2021; Hanna et al., 2021).

Models of grieving

Elisabeth Kübler-Ross (1969) theorises that grief can be segmented into five stages: denial, anger, bargaining, depression, and acceptance. Denial, as an initial reaction,

DOI: 10.4324/9781032660912-4

represents the reflection of a false reality, in which the terminally ill patient prefers to cling, believing that the diagnosis is false or somehow mistaken. Denial was considered predominantly harmful in the past, while more recent research suggests that denial may offer protection from unnecessary pain, but this may become unhealthy if it remains a constant state of mind (Janoff-Bulman, 1992). Anger is the stage of recognition by the individual that denial cannot continue and marks a return from the 'preferable' into the 'actual' reality. Bargaining revolves around the hope that the reason of grief can be exchanged, usually for a reformed way of life or seeking a compromise. This stage can also be interpreted as a phase of false hope. Depression is a stage of recognition of the individual's mortality, being a feeling of 'living in the present', surrounded often by emptiness, due to an upcoming loss that is inevitable. Acceptance as a final stage represents the embrace of an inevitable future, a stable condition of emotions, a calm retrospective of the individual, where the people dying might precede in this state the survivors (Kübler-Ross, 1969).

The Kübler-Ross model has been criticised for a lack of empirical evidence. Furthermore, the model is a product of a certain time and certain people, which may not be transferable to all contexts. Originally developed to describe what patients go through when dealing with a terminal illness, the model has been only applied later to grieving family members, who seemed to undergo a similar process. Even Kübler-Ross denied that grief would follow a linear pathway through all the five stages (Kübler-Ross and Kessler, 2005). Other studies suggest that experiencing grief is very subjective, sometimes experiencing one or more of the stages, repeating or skipping some of them, other times rushing through all of them or going through stages that were never part of the initial model (Shermer, 2008; Tang and Chow, 2017).

The work of Zisook and Shear (2009) suggests that there could be four major components of grief that manifest in different forms depending on the individual and the unique circumstances of the loss. First, separation distress represents a group of feelings including sadness, anxiety, pain, helplessness, shame, anger, or loneliness; traumatic distress, a group that includes states of disbelief and shock, intrusions, and efforts to avoid the emotions produced by this intrusion; guilt, remorse, and regrets and finally, social withdrawal. Zisook and Shear (2009) suggest that there is an instinctive path that grief takes that leads to better outcomes, called 'acute grief'. Those who suffer for longer periods of time may be experiencing a block of that pathway, known as 'prolonged or complex grief'. While some people will experience moderate feelings of sadness even after longer periods of time since the loss of a loved one, 'acute grief' will lessen within a few months. 'Prolonged grief' may often look like depression, and usually requires counselling or other kind of treatments (Szanto et al., 2006). 'Prolonged grief' can also be complicated by substance abuse, to escape some of the pain caused by grief, which can make coping even more complex (Shear and Mulhare, 2008).

Another model of grief developed by Corless (2010) describes three distinctive stages, including: notification and shock, experiencing the loss, and reintegration. During the first stage, the individual acknowledges or first learns about the loss, often isolating themselves from others, as the feeling of shock and numbness overwhelms. In the second stage, the loss is experienced both emotionally and cognitively, inducing feelings of anger, sadness, emptiness, or even physical manifestations such as sleep or eating disorders (Lowey, 2008). The final stage is when the individual returns, reorganizes, and reintegrates into their life, accepting the loss, carrying on without them. At this last stage, ideally the healing should take place at the end of grief (Corless, 2010). The key stages of the models of grieving discussed above are summarised in Table 4.1.

Vachon (2001), described nurses as wounded healers. While at the heart of the relationship between nurses and patients, caring and compassion positively affects patient care, "caring might come with a cost" (Boyle, 2011; Lally, 2005). Unacknowledged grief, if not recognising and coping with it, may escalate further, 'taking its toll' at a later stage (Wakefield, 2000). Compassion fatigue may be another consequence of caring for suffering patients. Compassion fatigue can be a result of nurses showing compassion while caring for patients who are dying or suffering daily (Austin et al., 2009). The effects of cumulative grief may cause compassion fatigue in nurses, who detach emotionally, or overinvest in patients' lives (Boyle, 2011). Unresolved cumulative grief and compassion fatigue can have consequences for an organisation in terms of increases in absenteeism, interpersonal and performance issues, decreased quality of patient care, and increased staff turnover (Aycock and Boyle, 2009; Showalter, 2010).

Understanding the complexity of the bereavement process and analysing and comparing different grieving models, although largely critiqued by their lack of empirical evidence, helped me acknowledging the existence of certain aspects discussed within these models in the empirical data of my research that formed the basis of this book.

Distancing and connecting emotionally

Coping strategies adopted by healthcare professionals (HCPs) after witnessing death and the management of the associated emotional labour have been widely researched. Avoidance, shielding, or objectification was often reported by HCPs, as an attempt to avoid distress, suffering, or the feelings of helplessness in cases when an emotional relationship was established with the dying patient and their

Table 4.1 Various models of grieving and their stages

Model of grieving	*Number of stages*	*Description*
Kübler-Ross	5	•Denial •Anger •Bargaining •Depression •Acceptance
Zisook and Shear	4	•Separation distress •Traumatic distress •Guilt, remorse, and regrets •Social withdrawal
Corless	3	•Acknowledging the loss •Experiencing the loss •Accepting the loss

family (Bailey et al., 2011a). Open conversations about death and the development of an emotional intelligence were positive strategies adopted by HCPs to help them deal with their experiences of death in the Emergency Department (ED). Witnessing death in the ED has an emotional impact on HCPs' wellbeing, who often developed strategies to protect themselves from the adverse effects of these experiences, as suggested by a study conducted in a UK hospital (Bailey et al., 2011b). Objectification, taking away the personhood of the deceased patient or avoidance, were means of HCPs to protect themselves from building a relationship that could potentially carry harmful effects for them, as one nurse described, "It's never someone, it's something in the viewing room. This is the language we use" (Bailey et al., 2011c). HCPs reported that the greatest challenge, when struggling with avoidance, comes from situations when someone is dying slowly (Bailey et al., 2011a). ED doctors often also expressed concerns about being emotionally attached to their end-of-life patients, as it could have an influence on their decision-making process, describing it as "(If) we are emotionally involved, it becomes hard to think in a clear minded way… I'm not entirely comfortable" (Yingting et al., 2018). A similar form of avoidance from HCPs towards the dying patient and their family manifests in concentrating on practical care tasks, sometimes 'shielding' and waiting for the patient to be potentially transferred, as being in their proximity gives staff a sense of discomfort (Di Leo et al., 2019). Avoiding conversations or meetings with relatives was another strategy adopted by clinical staff to protect themselves from the dead body becoming 'real' (Bailey et al., 2011a, c). Finding the 'right' balance between staying close or distancing from a dying patient creates a feeling of 'uneasiness' in HCPs when caring for a dying patient. As a member of staff suggested, "Sometimes we shield ourselves behind the fact we're busy carrying out our work", avoidance was used as an escape from building an empathetic relationship, to prevent becoming upset when death occurs (Di Leo et al., 2019).

Medical students interviewed in a Lebanese study also reported that HCPs working in the ED were looking to distance themselves and detach from the dying patients, as a way of softening the emotional impact, often labelled as a 'form of defence mechanism', while others were seeking to follow a task-oriented strategy. Some participants stated that experiencing 'the worst' helps in adapting and coping better with future deaths. Emotion-focused coping was also seen by clinical staff as a learning experience, which helped them to become less attached, more confident, or 'expecting the worst' (Batley et al., 2017). Individual reactions and the extent of the emotional effects of witnessing death in the ED are often related to factors including the patient's age, the expectation or suddenness of death, the level of relationship with the patient and their families, and the visibility of a family member's reactions (Batley et al., 2017). Overall emotional reactions of HCPs were also influenced by the coping mechanisms adopted, if the death witnessed was the first ever experienced, and if the death was relatable to personal experiences (Batley et al., 2017). Medical students interviewed described death on wards as impactful, due to the high level of interaction with patients and their families, in comparison the deaths in the ED which were also described as impactful but because of the added trauma, disturbing imagery and emotionally moving family reactions (Batley et al., 2017). The words used to describe the death experience on the ward included grief, sadness, feeling heartbroken and upset, compared with ED which used words such as shock, confusion, and surprise (Batley et al., 2017).

ED nurses interviewed in a Spanish study reported that they express feelings of helplessness, distress, suffering, and even anger when trying to act as advocates on behalf of the end-of-life patients, often confronting doctors who may treat the patient only based on pathological and clinical aspects (Jimenez-Herrera and Axelsson, 2015). More than 200 emergency nurses surveyed by Giles et al. (2019), and 43 emergency and palliative nurses surveyed and interviewed by Peters et al. (2013) reported that witnessing 'large scale' trauma events, such as a major accident, compared to repeatedly witnessing 'small scale' situations, can potentially have the same emotional influence on them, suggesting that repeated exposure to minor traumatising events can have severe consequences. ED nurses described 'feeling guilty' from not spending more time with dying patients and their families, or not meeting their end-of-life needs (Peters et al., 2013). Some nurses reported that "this feeling stays with you" or expressed their frustration because "not the right care was given" (Giles et al., 2019).

When emergency and palliative nurses coping mechanisms were compared, ED nurses consistently reported significantly lower coping regarding dealing with a dying patient and the family members, due to the nature of sudden and unexpected death (Peters et al., 2013). Dealing with grief and emotional issues surrounding death in the ED environment and during the little time available, was reported by emergency nurses as offering minimal opportunities to cope. ED nurses experiencing unexpected and traumatic patient deaths reported difficulties finding the words to speak with families of dying patients, especially when increased workloads and time pressure is present. Nurses with longer clinical experience, on the other hand, showed significantly higher coping skills compared to their less experienced colleagues (Peters et al., 2013). An Australian study among HCPs working in the ED found that despite the complex emotional effects of the death experience on them, HCPs mostly agreed that "caring for a dying patient in the ED is a reasonable demand on them". Most of them agreed that "it is rewarding caring for a dying patient", although many concluded that the ED is "not the right place to die" (Marck et al., 2014).

Managing emotional labour is required in coping with the influence of death. Emotional labour that accompanies a critical event in the ED can be described as demanding, an attitude that requires sensitivity when acting and reacting in a traumatic situation (Bailey et al., 2011a). Hochschild (1983) defines emotional labour as "the induction or suppression of feeling to sustain an outward appearance that produces in others a sense of being cared for in a convivial, safe place". Emotional intelligence has four major components such as self-awareness, self-management, social awareness, and relationship management, which allows HCPs working in the ED to recognise other individuals' emotions and regulate their own. This requires using 'gut feeling' or intuition to guide decisions and actions (Bailey et al., 2011c).

Self-awareness allows HCPs to identify strengths and weaknesses in their practice, reflect on and learn from past experiences while integrating core values into practice. Self-management involves the control of emotions in response to a traumatic event or a highly demanding work environment (Bailey et al., 2011c). The ability to demonstrate self-control in potentially emotionally intense situations is not directly proportional with the number of years spent in the ED by HCPs (Bailey et al., 2011c). Social awareness relates to the ability to understand another person's emotions, interpret, and communicate within social networks, for example, when an ED nurse, despite time pressures, can prioritise a dying patient and their family's needs and wishes. Relationship management requires skills to manage conflicts as well as to be an inspiration, motivation, and source of development for others. Developing emotional intelligence could potentially help HCPs in providing self-support, especially during traumatising events (Bailey et al., 2011c). The four major components of emotional intelligence are represented in Figure 4.1.

ED nurses have clearly identified a link between caring for terminally ill patients, patients transitioning from active treatment into palliative care, and patients being in pain and emotional labour. ED nurses who are unable to manage this emotional labour will most likely adopt a distancing behaviour to protect themselves from grief, although this coping mechanism can be more stressful for most nurses in the long term (Bailey et al., 2011c). Nurses reporting an inability to engage in emotional labour suggested that this was due to personal anxieties over death, being unable to handle their own feelings in a traumatic situation, fears of saying or doing the wrong thing, and the feeling of being untrained or unprepared when sudden death of a patient occurred (Bailey et al., 2011c). While further research is still required for evidence, a possible link could be observed between not being able to

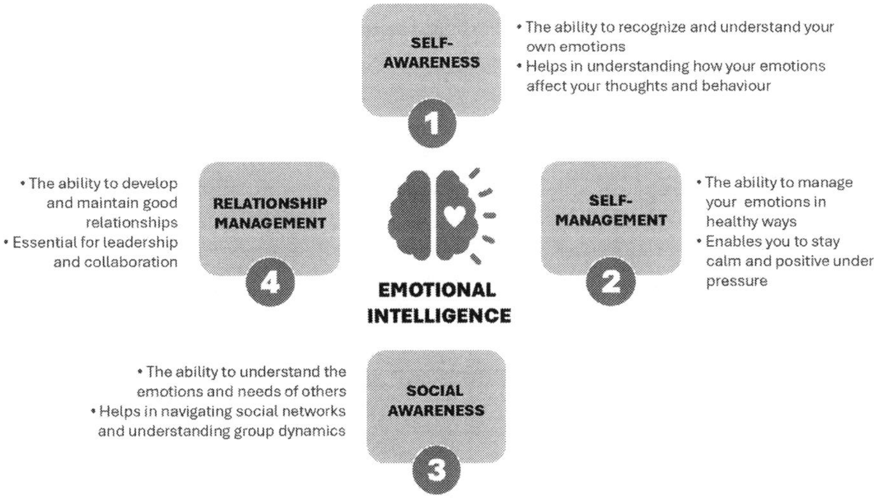

Figure 4.1 The four components of emotional intelligence.

manage emotional labour, resulting from managing death in an ED environment, and leaving emergency nursing as a profession. Experiences with dying patients were described by some nurses as overwhelming events, with heavy emotional impact on their professional role and often on their personal life. However, ED nurses demonstrate countless times, the ability to develop emotional intelligence, as a method of self-support that relies on their inner resources, to solve problems, facilitate learning, and manage change (Bailey et al., 2011a).

Support with managing death and dying

Dignity, relationships with end-of-life patients and their families, coping mechanisms, and emotional labour in relation to the death experience in the ED are better managed by HCPs when they develop resilience through support from their supervisors. This may be provided by staffing adequate skill-mix on shifts, through debriefs, or through receiving tailored training about managing the death experience. HCPs often feel unprepared for caring for the dying patient, partly because of the lack of support from managers in providing adequate professional training to address the issues raised by these experiences. As a result, staff rely on learning from others and from their own experience (Bailey et al., 2011c). Support should not start in the ED, but earlier, in undergraduate and postgraduate education. At undergraduate level, the focus should be on the effect of end-of-life care delivery in critical care areas and building awareness of the psychological and emotional needs of both staff and patients. At postgraduate level, supportive practice for trained staff and acknowledgement of their role and understanding how to manage the emotional impact in the end-of-life care delivery are the key elements for doctors and nurses working in the ED, to feel prepared in their roles (Bailey et al., 2011a).

Education and professional training are an efficient tool in supporting ED HCPs, not only to cope with the consequences of traumatising events, but also to facilitate conversations about dignity in the ED. Specialised training that would equip HCPs with such knowledge would provide additional support in decision-making and managing their own feelings in relation to death and dying (Mar Díaz-Cortés et al., 2018). In a similar way, education promoting professional development of efficient communication skills with the dying patient and their family is widely considered valuable elements of providing support for HCPs. According to nurses, "[We need] education sessions outlining strategies when dealing with patients and families", rationalising that training sessions could offer greater confidence to staff to comply with the demanding role of carrying for end-of-life patients (Peters et al., 2013). Education concerning counselling, delivering bad news, or conducting difficult conversations is considered by HCPs as an indispensable support in the ED (Giles et al., 2019). According to a study conducted in a US hospital, managers and administrators ensuring appropriate staffing rates, a good mix of knowledge, skills, and expertise during shifts, at any given time, will support the delivery and will positively influence the care provided for the dying patient (Chan, 2011). Several studies have reported on the importance of debriefs, as means in supporting HCPs with managing their death experiences, and as being an efficient way to cope with a failed resuscitation or a traumatic event. However, these are often missed or postponed due to time pressures (Giles et al., 2019; Peters et al., 2013). It is often common practice for debriefs to be organised several days or weeks after the incident, often led by facilitators with no expertise, perceived by many HCPs working in the ED as unhelpful (Giles et al., 2019). However, some emergency nurses argued that debriefs are not required after each death event, a formal debrief should be only conducted in special circumstances, such as the death of a child or in case of a traumatic death. While many nurses had to organise their own informal debrief with colleagues, it has been recognised that more regular and consistent debriefing would positively impact the provision of end-of-life care in the ED (Giles et al., 2019). Any form of professional support offered to staff appears to have a very positive impact on successfully managing the death and dying experience in an ED environment, leading to an increase in job satisfaction among clinical staff in general (Bailey et al., 2011b, c).

Reference list

Austin, W., Goble, E., Leier, B., Byrne, P. (2009). Compassion fatigue: The experience of nurses. *Ethics and Social Welfare*, 3(2), pp. 195–214.

Aycock, N., Boyle, D. (2009). Interventions to manage compassion fatigue in oncology nursing. *Clinical Journal of Oncology Nursing*, 13(2), pp. 183–191.

Bailey, C., Murphy, R., Porock, D. (2011a). Trajectories of end-of-life care in the emergency department. *Annals of Emergency Medicine*, 57(4), pp. 362–369.

Bailey, C., Murphy, R., Porock, D. (2011b). Dying cases in emergency places: Caring for the dying in emergency departments. *Social Science and Medicine*, 73(9), pp. 1371–1377.

Bailey, C., Murphy, R., Porock, D. (2011c). Professional tears: Developing emotional intelligence around death and dying in emergency work. *Journal of Clinical Nursing*, 20(23–24), pp. 3364–3372.

Batley, N.J., Bakhti, R., Chami, A., Jabbour, E., Bachir, R., El Khuri, C., Mufarrij, A.J. (2017). The effect of patient death on medical students in the emergency department. *BMC Medical Education*, 17(1), p. 110.

Boyle, D.A. (2011). Countering compassion fatigue: A requisite nursing agenda. *Online Journal of Issues in Nursing*, 16(1), pp. 1–16.

Chan, G.K. (2011). Trajectories of approaching death in the Emergency Department: Clinician narratives of patient transitions to the end of life. *Journal of Pain and Symptom Management*, 42(6), pp. 864–881.

Corless, I.B. (2010). *Oxford textbook of palliative nursing*. New York: Oxford University Press.

Das, S., Singh, T., Varma, R., Arya, Y.K. (2021). Death and mourning process in frontline health care professionals and their families during COVID-19. *Frontiers in Psychiatry*, 12, p. 624428.

Di Leo, S., Alquati, S., Autelitano, C., Costantini, M., Martucci, G., De Vincenzo, F., Kuczynska, B., Morini, A., Trabucco, L., Ursicelli, R., Catania, G., Ghirotto, L. (2019). Palliative care in the emergency department as seen by providers and users: a qualitative study. *Scandinavian Journal of Trauma, Resuscitation and Emergency Medicine*, 27, p. 88. Available at: https://doi.org/10.1186/s13049-019-0662-y

Giles, T.M., Hammad, K., Breaden, K., Drummond, C., Bradley, S.L., Gerace, A., Muir-Cochrane, E. (2019). Nurses' perceptions and experiences of caring for patients who die in the emergency department setting. *International Emergency Nursing*, 47, p. 100789. Available at: https://pubmed.ncbi.nlm.nih.gov/31495727

Hanna, J.R., Rapa, E., Dalton, L.J., Hughes, R., Quarmby, L.M., McGlinchey, T., Donnellan, W.J., Bennett, K.M., Mayland, C.R., Mason, S.R. (2021). Health and social care professionals' experiences of providing end of life care during the COVID-19 pandemic: A qualitative study. *Palliative Medicine*, 35(7), pp. 1249–1257.

Hochschild, A.R. (1983). *The managed heart. Commercialization of human feeling*. Berkeley: University of California Press.

Howarth, G. (2007). *Death and dying. A sociological introduction*. Cambridge: Polity Press.

Janoff-Bulman, R. (1992). *Shattered assumptions. Towards a new psychology of trauma*. New York: The Free Press.

Jimenez-Herrera, M.F., Axelsson, C. (2015). Some ethical conflicts in emergency care. *Nursing Ethics*, 22(5), pp. 548–560.

Kaplow, J.B., Saunders, J., Angold, A., Costello, E.J. (2010). Psychiatric symptoms in bereaved versus non-bereaved youth and young adults: A longitudinal epidemiological study. *Journal of the American Academy of Child and Adolescent Psychiatry*, 49(11), pp. 1145–1154.

Kübler-Ross, E. (1969). *On death and dying*. New York: The Macmillan Company.

Kübler-Ross, E., Kessler, D. (2005). *On grief and grieving. Finding the meaning of grief through the five stages of loss*. New York: Scribner.

Lally, R. (2005). Oncology nurses share their experiences with bereavement and self-care. *ONS News*, 20(10), pp. 4–11.

Lowey, S.E. (2008). Letting go before a death: A concept analysis. *Journal of Advanced Nursing*, 63(2), pp. 208–215.

Mar Díaz-Cortés, M.D., Granero-Molina, J., Hernández-Padilla, J.M., Rodríguez, R.P., Casado, M.C., Fernández-Sola, C. (2018). Promoting dignified end-of-life care in the emergency department: A qualitative study, *International Emergency Nursing*, 37, pp. 23–28.

Marck, C.H., Weil, J., Lane, H., Weiland, T.J., Philip, J., Boughey, M., Jelinek, G.A. (2014). Care of the dying cancer patient in the emergency department: Findings from a National survey of Australian emergency department clinicians. *Internal Medicine Journal*, 44(4), pp. 362–368.

Morris, S. (2011). The psychology of grief – Applying cognitive and behaviour therapy principles. *InPsych*, 33(6). Available at: https://psychology.org.au/for-members/publications/inpsych/2011/dec/the-psychology-of-grief-applying-cognitive-and-b (Accessed: 18 April 2024).

Newson, R.S., Boelen, P.A., Hek, K., Hofman, A., Tiemeier, H. (2011). The prevalence and characteristics of complicated grief in older adults. *Journal of Affective Disorders*, 132(1–2), pp. 231–238.

Peters, L., Cant, R., Payne, S., O'Connor, M., McDermott, F., Hood, K., Morphet, J., Shimoinaba, K. (2013). Emergency and palliative care nurses' levels of anxiety about death and coping with death: A questionnaire survey. *Australasian Emergency Nursing Journal*, 16(4), pp. 152–159.

Schoenberger, J.M., Yeghiazarian, S., Rios, C., Henderson, S.O. (2013). Death notification in the Emergency Department: Survivors and physicians. *Western Journal of Emergency Medicine*, 15(2), pp. 181–185.

Shear, M.K., Mulhare, E. (2008). Complicated grief. *Psychiatric Annals*, 38(10), pp. 662–670.

Shermer, M. (2008). *Five fallacies of grief: Debunking psychological stages*. Available at: https://www.scientificamerican.com/article/five-fallacies-of-grief/ (Accessed: 05 July 2024).

Showalter, S.E. (2010). Compassion fatigue: What is it? Why does it matter? Recognizing the symptoms, acknowledging the impact, developing the tools to prevent compassion fatigue, and strengthen the professional already suffering from the effects. *American Journal of Hospice and Palliative Medicine*, 27(4), pp. 239–242.

Szanto, K., Shear, M.K., Houck, P.R. (2006). Indirect self-destructive behaviour and overt suicidality in patients with complicated grief. *Journal of Clinical Psychiatry*, 67(2), pp. 233–239.

Tang, S., Chow, A.Y.M. (2017). Subjective and objective traumatic death: Distinct roles in developing complicated grief and depression among older adults in Hong Kong. *International Psychogeriatrics*, 29(3), pp. 409–417.

Torrens-Burton, A., Goss, S. Sutton, E., Barawi, K., Longo, M., Seddon, K., Carduff, E., Farnell, D.J.J., Nelson, A., Byrne, A., Phillips, R., Selman, L.E., Harrop, E. (2022). 'It was brutal. It still is': A qualitative analysis of the challenges of bereavement during the COVID-19 pandemic reported in two national surveys. *Palliative Care and Social Practice*, 16. Available at: https://doi.org/10.1177/26323524221092456 (Accessed: 05 May 2024).

Yingting, Z., Yash Pal, R., Wai, T., Wilson, S., Lee, A., Ong, M., Hwaa, T.L. (2018). Spiritual perspectives of emergency medicine doctors and nurses in caring for end-of-life patients: A mixed-method study. *International Emergency Nursing*, 37, pp. 13–22.

Zisook, S., Shear, K. (2009). Grief and bereavement: What psychiatrists need to know. *World Psychiatry*, 8(2), pp. 67–74.

Vachon, M.L. (2001). *Textbook of palliative care nursing*. New York: Oxford University Press.

Wakefield, A. (2000). Nurses' responses to death and dying: A need for relentless self-care. *International Journal of Palliative Nursing*, 6(5), pp. 245–251.

Wallace, C.L., Wladkowski, S.P., Gibson, A., White, P. (2020). Grief during the COVID-19 pandemic: Considerations for palliative care providers. *Journal of Pain and Symptom Management*, 60(1), pp. 70–76.

Chapter 5

Experiencing death in the Emergency Department

One of the important observations drawn from the individual conversations with participants of my study was that everyone is 'carrying' certain experiences, as 'lasting memories' of death cases in the Emergency Department (ED). Exploring and understanding the characteristics of these cases, trying to find the answer to the question, why some deaths become unforgettable, what makes them so unique, that they leave a lasting impression on healthcare professionals (HCPs) is one of the aspects of the death experience, this chapter will cover. The other aspect endeavours to understand when and how the objectification of patients, who require a life-saving intervention, could happen in the ED, and how the cultural and social background of the patient, together with the impact that the grieving family members can have on staff, influences the death and dying experience.

Emergency Department deaths to remember

Participants of the study talked about witnessing death in the ED on a regular basis, on average at least once over a week period, depending on their shift pattern and time spent in the Resuscitation Room (Resus), where most deaths occur. Although this constant exposure to death caused most of the participants to 'get used' to this experience, all participants could recall cases that were 'memorable' for them. Some of the participants expressed during the interviews that they did not have to think which one to choose, as particular deaths 'stuck with them'. When asked about what specific features make a death memorable, the most common characteristics described were a child or young adult death; traumatic, sudden, unexpected, or shocking death; death that occurred during the early career or those that resembles a similarity with the death of a family member.

> Probably one of the daunting ones is one that I have broken down after, was an auntie who was walking her nephew and niece home from school and the nephew was in a pushchair and the niece was on a scooter. They've reached a zebra crossing where a car stopped and the little girl went forward, but they haven't seen that there was a motorbike coming and hit her headfirst. She came in as a traumatic cardiac arrest and I was looking to this little girl while they

DOI: 10.4324/9781032660912-5

> were doing CPR, cannulatc, taking bloods, who has donc nothing wrong in her life and is just hanging to life. She passed away and it was horrific because the parents weren't there, only her auntie.
>
> (Julie, Healthcare Assistant)

> There are a couple that stick with me. Quite a lot of paediatric ones that I always think about, quite frequently... I think we had a 5-month old that drowned in a swimming pool and it was under the supervision of his brother who was 17 or 18, and he found him after 20 minutes in the swimming pool face down in the evening ... in a couple of minutes we had another call which was a 6-month old, who was septic and arrested, and we had those both in the bays side by side due to logistics really... That is something that stuck with me.
>
> (Robert, Advanced Clinical Practitioner)

The cases that were described as 'daunting', 'horrific', 'emotional', or 'really hard' are often the direct triggers to feelings of helplessness, arising from the inability to change the outcome. In the process of coming to terms with the death of a child, many individuals find themselves searching for a deeper meaning or rationale to help make sense of such a profound loss. This search for meaning can be an important part of the grieving and acceptance journey, offering a way to cope with the overwhelming emotions that accompany such a tragedy. Often, people reflect on the inherent vulnerability and delicate nature of children, recognizing how their physical and emotional fragility can make them more susceptible to harm compared to adults.

Moreover, another deeply distressing aspect of a child's death is the emotional toll it takes on the parents. It raises questions about how they will navigate life after such a loss, how they will find the strength to move forward, and how they will cope with the absence of someone who was so central to their world. The grief is not only about the life that was lost but also about the future that will never be realized, making the mourning process uniquely painful and complex.

A child's death was often linked by the study participants to a moral duty and an ethical responsibility, that somehow, they 'had to do something' to save that life. Other times the death of a child leaves a void, a feeling of emptiness, by 'not knowing what to do', often avoiding facing their own personal feelings after the event.

> Every child case will be emotional, but this was the only one where the child was alive at arrival. A child arrives alive they shouldn't die, as it should be something we could do. I guess the emotional toll of this is harder ... you still feel that you should have done something.
>
> (Andrew, Consultant)

A death that features traumatic characteristics, accompanied by powerful visual elements, often involving the loss of a high volume of blood or other bodily fluids, a severe deformity of parts of the body, a rapid and sudden deterioration, sometimes followed by the patient's verbal and non-verbal reactions, has been accounted by participants as particular cases to remember. A sense of helplessness in such cases among participants, not being able to fulfil their life-saving aim, was very frequent.

> There is another one which is awful, it was a guy with oesophageal cancer, it ruptured some oesophageal varices, and he was bleeding out, so coughing up blood, swallowing blood, vomiting blood and conscious at the same time. And he had metastases everywhere. I remember seeing him in the ED and just knowing, that there is nothing we could actually do for him. That was just the most awful visual experience.
>
> (Robert, Advanced Clinical Practitioner)

Erica, one of the members of staff, who had less than a year of experience in the ED at the time of the interviews, and had started there as a newly qualified nurse, said that she had never lost anyone close to her, in her family or circle of friends. She witnessed her first death in the ED, this lack of previous exposure making this death a shocking experience.

> There was a lot of blood, and I was in some kind of shock as I have never seen anything like that before, I have never seen anyone dead, so it was like … I have never seen a case as a nurse where they don't survive. So, it was really bizarre that we are just leaving it and walking away.
>
> (Erica, Nurse)

Death experienced during the early career period, especially if the case resembles traumatic or visually disturbing features, can contribute to being described as 'awful' and 'horrible'. Nicholas describes one of his memorable deaths from his early years in practice, as a traumatic death of a patient who was 'making eye-contact' with him while actively dying.

> There is definitely one that I had, which sticks with me since I was F1 or F2, a very junior doctor … There was this patient that we never met before, didn't knew anything about him and was having faecal vomit … In essence, this guy, unfortunately was vomiting so much, that he chocked, on his own vomit … We've tried very hard to keep him alive and it took him 20–30 minutes to die in his own vomit, which at that time, being an F1, was a horrible experience as he was making eye contact with me while he was going and going, and he had glassier eye. It was awful.
>
> (Nicholas, Consultant)

Most participants gave accounts about experiencing death in their personal life, prior to start working in the ED, and how that affected them. While some suggested that they were not reminded by these deaths while working, others often spotted a similarity with a deceased relative or even themselves. A similar age, physical features, or the medical condition of the patient, could make these cases feel connected to a personal experience, tapping into personal fears for the self or for loved ones.

> Since my mum died, I notice more similarities. Especially when cases are similar. When there is a patient of similar age or similar diagnosis. She was a terminal cancer case that was diagnosed very late.
>
> (Isaac, Charge Nurse)

> For example, we had a cardiac arrest in Resus. Young, 47-year old and I was thinking, this could be me.
>
> (Zoe, Senior Sister)

Participants often expressed their feelings of being more empathetic towards dying patients and their families, when there is a similarity that reminds them of someone close to them, such as a parent or a sibling, or a particular case when someone close to them died.

> If the patient is your personal age, like the other day there was a patient, very similar age to me, so you make the connection … that's me. Then if it's my parents' age I connect them with my parents. For example, we had a patient passing away, her sister came in saying 'Please don't let her die, we are best friends.' You see, I've got a twin sister, you empathize in that respect.
>
> (Margaret, Sister)

> Back in the days I was working as a nanny, and I was looking after a child for 8 months who died and that was killing me. And when this mother said, nobody understands what it means to lose a child, this is what I was thinking, that it wasn't biologically mine, but it felt like it was mine.
>
> (Julie, Healthcare Assistant)

Participants talked about a substantial difference between a death that can be anticipated, in comparison to the one that occurs without any warning. These sudden and unexpected deaths become memorable because often staff establishes a relationship with the patient, they build a rapport, determine a course of action or treatments before they die. These outcomes, which suddenly deviate from the original plan and the purpose of their role, are seen as shocking and are interpreted as impacting significantly on participants.

> He had quite a few comorbidities and he had full-time carers. I had a bit of a rapport with him. Unfortunately, he suddenly arrested, which although he was

> unwell, he wasn't looking that unwell. It was quite a shock, I guess and obviously we've tried everything we could to bring him back, but unfortunately, he died.
>
> (Rachel, Advanced Clinical Practitioner)

> I think the ones that made the most significant impact for me were those who, I wouldn't say were clinically well at the time, but I had an interaction, a bit of rapport and they suddenly deteriorated, I think those are the ones that stick with me the most … when it's really unexpected and out-of-the-blue and that's when it's difficult.
>
> (Charlie, Healthcare Assistant)

A sudden death was often connected by participants to the age of the deceased patient and the general expectation that comes with it. A young and active person is not expected to die, in comparison with someone nearing to the end of their natural life. Personal values of participants were often reflected in these accounts, referring to some of these deaths as being 'acceptable' or quite the opposite.

> These ones are less predictable to end in a death, they are much more unexpected … Young people, being more active, not being at the end of their natural life, I guess makes it more memorable, compared to the ninety years old coming from a nursing home with a cardiac arrest, it's even more acceptable, isn't it? I know it sounds horrible, but compared to someone who is thirty weeks pregnant that is not someone coming to the end of their life. That is exactly the opposite.
>
> (Isaac, Charge Nurse)

Some participants often described deaths becoming shocking to them, due to their randomness, and inability to find a meaning or a sense in them. As participants considered that some of these deaths could have been probably avoided, this made these deaths hard to understand or 'resonate' with them.

> It was this lady in her seventies, she was an antique's dealer, she was just shopping on a Saturday morning, was driving home and for whatever reason she was on the wrong side of the road and hit another car head on, but they think she might have had a stroke at the wheel … There was a man in his early seventies, but had advanced dementia, and he choked to death on a sausage … Then young people coming in with brain haemorrhages, they are fine, then they have a headache, you just see such a wide range … there are these ones that resonate with you.
>
> (Margaret, Sister)

Some of the deaths experienced by HCPs could combine a series of memorable features, including young age, severe trauma, and being unexpected, often referred to by participants as being 'horrific' or 'horrible'. Another reason for a death becoming memorable is when the treatment intervention is 'spectacular' and draws a lot of attention, such as a thoracotomy, or opening a patient's chest, caused, for example, by a penetrating cardiac trauma. Witnessing these deaths will often cause participants to feel upset or sad.

> Then I think it's a lot of the brutal ones that stick with you. We are a major trauma centre so we can crack-open people's chest.
>
> (Zoe, Senior Sister)

> But then you also see, the horrific, the horrible deaths that don't make you feel warm inside, but upset and sad. So earlier this year there was an 18-year-old girl who was in a boat crush, and she came in very poorly and despite everything we did, we couldn't save her. And her dad was the one that decided to stop the treatment. We said we can do this … but she would be either very disabled or brain damaged. The dad told us: 'I don't want that for my daughter, can we please stop treatment?' … so sadly she passed away … so that is one that will stay with me forever. It was sad.
>
> (Margaret, Sister)

Objectifying and humanising death

Death can be a complex experience in the ED, where patients sometimes could be objectified and later humanised again. This experience is often characterised by providing care and life-saving treatment in an 'autopilot mode' or when death 'becomes personal' by discovering the person behind the patient, through communication with the family or through learning about their social and cultural background. Many participants of the study described their 'natural' way of dealing with a patient being in a life-threatening condition, as an 'autopilot mode'. This describes a highly alerted and very focused state of the mind when all effort is put into saving the patient's life. Technical skills are prioritised, such as resuscitation techniques and often an 'objectification' of the individual happens, to increase efficiency. This state is usually maintained until either the patient resuscitation is successful, fails, or a decision is made to stop. Participants described following a 'script', an 'algorithm', or a 'protocol' during resuscitation as making them feel being less exposed emotionally to the situation.

> Because when they come in arrested, you just automatically focus on the patient and there are no emotions there, you just automatically have to save their life … I think we just have to save this patient's life, and sometimes we just go into action, as in auto-pilot mode, because this is what you are trained to do.
>
> (Zoe, Senior Sister)

> You know we have some people who are extremely clinical, we come together as the patient is almost an object, let's do this, let's do that, everything is structured but when it comes to the holistic side of things, it all goes out of the window.
>
> (Charlie, Healthcare Assistant)

> I remember once I was doing chest compressions on a 4-year-old and the family was there, and obviously the family was very emotional and screaming. And I was thinking, all I am concentrating on right now, is to make sure I am doing the depths of the chest compressions right … I knew my job was to do this, I was very focused on doing that. In those situations, I am fine, I am very good in focusing on the actual practical things rather than the emotional part of it.
>
> (David, Senior Charge Nurse)

Once resuscitation stops and the patient is declared dead, with family members being present or often arriving later, participants described this state as a quick, sudden transition from seeing the individual as a 'patient', into seeing them as a 'person'. The catalysts for this transition are often the family members, who through the after-death conversations will humanise the deceased. This transition was often described by participants as being difficult.

> I knew that's going to be difficult when they arrive and it was because suddenly you go from a professional, not lack of emotions, but a professional, as 'we are going to tick these boxes; we are going to make sure to address everything we can'. And suddenly this person arrives who is a human being, with feelings and I remember that being incredibly difficult.
>
> (Robert, Advanced Clinical Practitioner)

> The only time I get upset probably is when I see the reactions of the family because that's when it really hits home about … ahh this is a family member and then I can put myself in their position. That is the only time when I can feel a bit of emotion.
>
> (Christine, Senior Sister)

Witnessing intense emotional reactions from family members while delivering the bad news to them could further develop the complexity of the death experience for HCPs. Some of these experiences were described by participants as being the most difficult parts of the bereavement process, contributing for that death to become memorable.

> We and the consultant who was running, went in to meet mum and dad, and we break the bad news, and the scream that came out from that mum's mouth, will stay with me forever. I've never heard a mum make that noise

> about her child. It's just awful to think about. It was probably the most shocking one that makes you feel sick ... It was about 2 years ago now, but it stays with me.
>
> (Christine, Senior Sister)

Beyond a combination of features that will make a death a difficult experience, according to participants of this study, intense reactions of the family members will add to the depths of that experience. At this stage the patient appears as part of a larger social structure, reflecting in the relationships presented or the stories told by relatives, where their death leaves a void or an emptiness.

> The worst part for me are the relatives when they are crying and mourning and shouting, all this expression of pain they have, this is the worst part for me.
>
> (Annabelle, Healthcare Assistant)

> So, I was just watching the chest compressions ... Then eventually, the consultant came in and kind of said that we need to stop. The parents were just sat there, and it was horrific as they were screaming.
>
> (Erica, Nurse)

> Dealing with the family is probably the hardest bit. When a person is dying and telling that to the family is probably the toughest bit.
>
> (William, Registrar)

Some participants described death not only as a biological process, but suggested that death occurs earlier, before the physical death, when the patient stops interacting or the person they used to be disappears. This description of 'social death' suggests that the individual is considered dead or non-existent, and experiences a loss of identity and connectiveness, and even the act of grieving can start before the actual biological death occurs.

> I have been criticised before saying this, but for me, people die as a person before they physically die, when they stop interacting with you and stop being the character you know. For me there is an emotional disconnect at that point, for me that person is gone, it become someone else or something else at that point. The mourning can start even before they die.
>
> (John, Junior Doctor)

Participants have acknowledged that dealing with death, mourning, and grieving can vary depending on the cultural background of the patient and their close family. Cultural awareness is important, as many aspects of grieving, displayed by family members, could feel alien, something that HCPs, especially born and raised in a Western society, does not feel used to or comfortable with. Reactions of the family members, depending on their cultural background can range from loud screaming or the gathering of a large crowd in the clinical area, to mourn their loved one.

> I had people who got very hysterical even they knew this is going to happen. Some are very cultural. One patient's relative, who passed away, just absolutely freaked out, hitting themselves, shouting at me, stuff like this. Or I had someone who grabbed me and put their hand over my mouth saying: 'Don't say it, don't say it.' Just a total hysterical reaction. Me and the senior sister were in there and we understand that in different cultures, certain generations do respond like this, for example hitting themselves as a sign of their grief, something that I have never actually seen before. It's been really bizarre.
>
> (Nicholas, Consultant)

> You had quite large families turning up of 20–30 people, it's difficult isn't it, for us in healthcare, in England specifically, culturally, we are a bit like, that is too much, that does not feel comfortable to us. We haven't worked in other countries, and we haven't experienced death there. In some places the whole village will turn up in a hospital if someone dies.
>
> (Robert, Advanced Clinical Practitioner)

Some deaths were memorable to participants because of being perceived as having a 'good death'. These deaths were perceived as dignified, because they conformed to societal and cultural definitions of a dignified death from their perspective, patient and family wishes were respected, family had the opportunity to say their goodbyes, pain and symptoms were kept under control, and all unnecessary treatment was avoided. Some participants even suggested that we always seem to look to death 'as a negative', while such positive way a death was managed should be role modelled, when achieved in the ED.

> There was a lady … we knew she's going to pass away quite soon. So, putting her on a hospital bed, making her comfortable, getting her pillows, keeping her warm, brushing her hair, making sure she's clean, giving her a freshen-up, these are the things we can do for her. Making sure she's not in pain, giving her a small amount of pain relief making sure, she's not suffering in any way. Turn the lights down, put her in a side room, making it quiet, maybe put on some music on, of that era, something that suits her, because obviously she can still hear you. Talk to her, hold her hands. Getting the relatives in … inform them, get them in as soon as we can, make sure they can sit with her. Offer them a cup of tea, give them all the information they need. Answer any question that they have, give them the written information they need. Make sure they are not alone and that they are comfortable, offer a spiritual or religious leader, should they need one. So, I think even in the ED we can make end-of-life care really good, and I have seen that myself and I have enjoyed it, maybe that's not the right word, but just being part of it.
>
> (Margaret, Sister)

> Last Wednesday we had a very good death in the department. The patient came in they were clearly dying, we didn't do anything unnecessary, the family were

in. I don't think we celebrate those things ... we don't celebrate death enough. It's always a negative, I think.

(Robert, Advanced Clinical Practitioner)

Discussion: experiencing death in the Emergency Department

A study of oncology care providers has found that greater exposure to death is directly associated with greater levels of stress (Whippen and Canellos, 1991). Results of a further study have shown that the three most distressing events emergency nurses are repeatedly confronted with are cot death, incidents involving children, and dealing with patients' relatives and family (De Clercq et al., 2011). Deaths that are shocking and unexpected by their nature are known to generate more distress and result in a deeper psychological trauma than natural, planned, or expected deaths (Jackson et al., 2005). Other studies reported that a large number of doctors who witnessed 'memorable deaths', including death of young patients, death that lacks dignity, or death of a patient where a strong personal relationship pre-exists, that death remains emotionally distressing, triggering strong reactions, including, but not limited to stress, guilt, feelings of numbness, and feeling upset (Linklater, 2010; Redinbaugh et al., 2003). Emergency doctors specifically report insomnia, fatigue, sadness, and disappointment after facing unexpected deaths (Redinbaugh et al., 2003; Meier et al., 2001).

Consistent with these findings, another study reported that 49% of the interviewed doctors, as a consequence of patient death, expressed distress or fear, while almost 12% reported symptoms of post-traumatic stress disorder (PTSD), with 30% experiencing symptoms of either re-experiencing, avoidance, and arousal in relation to death (Mills and Mills, 2005). Factors that influence the intensity level of these emotional reactions include the age of the patient, cause of death, and presence of the family (Strote et al., 2011). These effects are also influenced by the level of training and years of experience a doctor has (Jackson et al., 2005). These findings are in line with another study which compared registered nurses' death anxiety and concluded that nurses' emotional distress was lower as age, education, and nursing experience increased (Deffner and Bell, 2005). One of the reasons a death in the ED has a significant influence on HCPs is when that occurs unexpectedly, is traumatic or have a rapid course, HCPs often not having the opportunity to prepare themselves emotionally for such events (Beckstrand et al., 2008). My empirical study similarly reports that the death of a child or young adult, a traumatic and unexpected death, a death that is witnessed by HCPs at the beginning of their career, or a death that displays a similarity between the deceased and themselves or a family member or friend had a considerable emotional and psychological influence on participants. The novelty of the findings is related to these specific experiences leaving a lasting impression, becoming memorable for HCPs, often described as being 'stuck with them'. The five major type of deaths in the ED that carries the possibility of becoming 'memorable' to HCPs are represented in Figure 5.1.

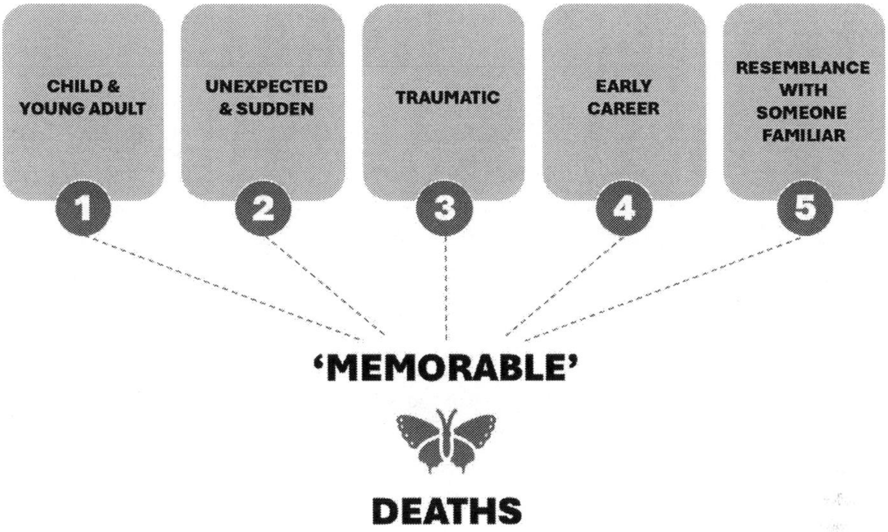

Figure 5.1 The five major type of deaths in the ED to leave a lasting impression on HCPs.

My empirical study reported that death in the ED can become a complex experience, requiring staff to suddenly transition from an 'autopilot' life-saving mode, into recognising the person behind the patient, particularly when interactions with the family are difficult or when death is accompanied by culture-specific reactions. A study investigating experiences of medical students, similarly, described their clinical work in critical situations, in the ED as 'autopilot mode', before meeting the family (Batley et al., 2017). Medical students referred to their emotional investment being less accentuated when performing cardiopulmonary resuscitation (CPR), or clinical interventions on dying patients, compared to when they'll meet the family of the deceased, and get to know the 'person', behind the 'patient'. This task-oriented approach often served as a defence strategy, against the feelings associated with death (Batley et al., 2017). Di Leo et al. (2019) similarly argues that whenever staff is concentrating on practical tasks, that involves a protection, a shielding from acknowledging the challenging emotions surrounding death. The same shielding from painful emotions was observed by Bailey et al. (2011a, b, c) in the ED nurses, in the form of using a language that avoids acknowledging the deceased patient as a 'person', referring to it only as a 'body', and an avoidance of meeting family members, in an attempt to stop the 'body' becoming 'real'. My study argues that the objectification of a patient does not only happen to protect HCPs from the emotional challenges surrounding death, yet often is a subconscious or even conscious decision during the resuscitation process, putting the emotional connectedness with the patient or the family aside, to follow an algorithm, aimed to save the patient's life. My research reaches to a similar conclusion, that often meeting family members, is the point when the 'objectified' patient is 'humanised' again.

Participants of my empirical study often talked about the cultural aspect of death, how for a HCP raised in a Western society, certain mourning rituals of family members, made them feel uncomfortable, or sometimes these even appear to be 'bizarre' expressions of grief. Participants interviewed often argued that learning about cultural-specific grieving rituals would help them better support families, especially when breaking the bad news. Family members can respond to the death notification of their loved one, in various ways, depending on a series of aspects, such as the patient's age, existing comorbidities, reason for commencing CPR, overall emotional state, spiritual norms, and cultural values, which impacts their attitudes towards death and dying (Naik, 2013). The cultural identity of an individual incorporates a series of elements, including self-identity, language, beliefs, traditions, religion, and their wider value system (Naik, 2013). Breaking the bad news to the family holds a higher risk of increased stress level and strong emotional reactions, when death is a result of a suicide, a criminal event, traffic accident, or when it is the death of a child (McClement et al., 2009). Roe (2012) makes a similar observation connecting adverse family reactions with the age of the patient, the opinion that the patient died prematurely, or the suddenness of death. Application of end-of-life strategy and bereavement care in the ED can be often limited by anger or agitation displayed by family members (Heaston et al., 2006).

A study of 11 Iranian nurses and doctors, from six hospitals, working in emergency or critical care, interviewed them about their experience with death notifications (Hassankhani et al., 2018). The study found that beyond the cause of resuscitation, the age of the patient, and the current emotional state of the family, ethnicity and cultural background plays an important role in what their reactions will be. The study acknowledges that Iran has a rich ethnic and cultural diversity, and each of them has their own individual death rituals and their unique attitudes towards the process of dying (Hassankhani et al., 2018). According to HCPs, the death of an older patient, whose death was expected, is accepted usually in a calm and quiet manner by family members, and communication is more efficient with those who have a 'non-aggressive' personality and higher education level. On the contrary, with certain cultural backgrounds, it is common to experience from family members, verbal or physical aggression towards hospital staff, and often severe emotional reactions such as screaming or self-harm (Hassankhani et al., 2018). Strategies adopted by staff to notify the family about the death of their loved one included talking softly and gently, using physical contact when appropriate, informing only the male members of the family, or talking with the wider circle of family only, allowing them to break the bad news with close family members, such as a parent or a spouse (Hassankhani et al., 2018). Participants of my empirical study often mentioned that Britain is a multi-cultural nation, and clinical staff can be exposed to unusual, unexpected, or extreme reactions from family members, during the death notification. Understanding the relationship between the grieving process and cultural characteristics is crucial in better preparing HCPs for the death and dying experience.

Participants in my study sometimes referred to death as something that happens even before the biological cessation of life, when the patient stops interacting, when they stop being the person they were before, and when an emotional disconnect surfaces. Sudnow (1967) described the term 'social death' as the moment from which the dying patient is considered by clinical staff as being 'already dead', surrounding him with a 'special treatment', which could include termination of active treatment or commencing of religious rites. Králová (2015) argues that social death can be described by three significant characteristics, which already compromised the individual's wellbeing: loss of social identity; loss of social connectedness; and losses associated with deformity or disintegration of the body. Lock (2002) suggests that experiencing social death involves someone undergoing a loss of moral entitlement. Another frequent example can be found in cases of cardiopulmonary resuscitation, when the perceived social value of a patient, regardless of the chances of survivability, influences a doctor's decisions to resuscitate (Timmermans, 1998). My study reflects on the experiences of HCPs, who sometimes consider a patient being 'already dead' when they cease to be the person they were before, or when they stop interacting. Decisions to continue resuscitation, being influenced by the social value of an individual, such as a child or young adult, were also confirmed by my study.

A crucial aspect related to the death and dying experience of clinical staff, the death notifier, the family of the deceased, and the recipient of the death notification is related to what were the circumstances of death and how the information is shared with the family (Adamowski et al., 1993; Stewart, 1999). Deaths that have sudden, traumatic, or even violent causes, including murder, suicide, road accidents, accidental overdose, or work-related severe injuries potentially have long-term effects of stress and discomfort on clinical staff (Marco and Wetzel, 2012; Hobgood et al., 2013). Similarly, family members who cannot find meaning in their traumatic experience, could be more exposed to experience long-term psychological distress, post-traumatic stress, and psychosomatic disorders (Neimeyer et al., 2002; Armour, 2003). Participants of my study, describing some of their death experiences as 'shocking' or 'horrifying', often triggered by the visual aspect of the dying process, described various physiological and psychological effects of these experiences, from difficulties sleeping, up to severe emotional distress.

Studies highlight the importance of death notification, especially if death had an unexpected, traumatic aspect, which if not done adequately, can have a significant influence on the bereavement process (Mitchell, 2008; Parris, 2011; Baumann and Stark, 2015). Tuffrey-Wijne and Rose (2017) argues that the psychological, physical, and social characteristics of the individuals who are going to be notified should be taken into consideration to evaluate potential health risks, for example, individuals with cognitive disabilities are often not notified of a death, being over-protected. The notification process is perceived by staff as a difficult and stressful event, especially in the light of shortage of educational material on how to deal with sudden death and how to handle painful communications in a sensitive, empathetic, respectful, and compassionate way (Smith et al., 1999; Ombres et al., 2017). Lack of training to facilitate preparation for the death and dying experience has been mentioned regularly by the participants of my study, discussed in more detail as part of the chapter 'The influence of death in the Emergency Department'.

This chapter concluded that the characteristics that make a death experience memorable for HCPs in the ED, often with a lasting impression even for decades, include the death of a child or young adult, a traumatic or sudden death, an early-career death, or a death of a patient that draws similarities to HCPs, with themselves or someone close to them. Objectification of a patient, as a measure of 'isolating emotionally' to better perform during the resuscitation of a patient, avoiding potential 'distractions' from a life-saving procedure, has also been discussed, alongside how humanising the same individual happens, when meeting members of their family.

Reference list

Adamowski, K., Dickinson, G., Weitzman, B., Roessler, C., Carter-Snell, C. (1993). Sudden unexpected death in the emergency department: Caring for the survivors. *Canadian Medical Association Journal*, 149(10), pp. 1445–1451.

Armour, M. (2003). Meaning making in the aftermath of homicide. *Death Studies*, 27(6), pp. 519–540.

Bailey, C., Murphy, R., Porock, D. (2011a). Trajectories of end-of-life care in the emergency department. *Annals of Emergency Medicine*, 57(4), pp. 362–369.

Bailey, C., Murphy, R., Porock, D. (2011b). Dying cases in emergency places: Caring for the dying in emergency departments. *Social Science and Medicine*, 73(9), pp. 1371–1377.

Bailey, C., Murphy, R., Porock, D. (2011c). Professional tears: developing emotional intelligence around death and dying in emergency work. *Journal of Clinical Nursing*, 20(23–24), pp. 3364–3372.

Batley, N.J., Bakhti, R., Chami, A., Jabbour, E., Bachir, R., El Khuri, C., Mufarrij, A.J. (2017). The effect of patient death on medical students in the emergency department. *BMC Medical Education*, 17(1), p. 110.

Baumann, R., Stark, S. (2015). The role of forensic death investigators interacting with the survivors of death by homicide and suicide. *Journal of Forensic Nursing*, 11(1), pp. 28–32.

Beckstrand, R., Smith, M.D., Heaston, S., Bond, A.E. (2008). Emergency nurses' perceptions of size, frequency, and magnitude of obstacles and supportive behaviours in end-of-life care. *Journal of Emergency Nursing*, 34(3), pp. 290–300.

De Clercq, F., Deheegher, J., Van Hoorde, H. (2011). Frequency of and subjective response to critical incidents in the prediction of PTSD in Emergency Personnel. *Journal of Traumatic Stress*, 24(1), pp. 133–136.

Deffner, J.M., Bell, S.K. (2005). Nurses' death anxiety, comfort level during communication with patients and families regarding death, and exposure to communication education: A quantitative study. *Journal of Nurses in Staff Development*, 21(1), pp. 19–23.

Di Leo, S., Alquati, S., Autelitano, C., Costantini, M., Martucci, G., De Vincenzo, F., Kuczynska, B., Morini, A., Trabucco, L., Ursicelli, R., Catania, G., Ghirotto, L. (2019). Palliative care in the emergency department as seen by providers and users: a qualitative study.

Scandinavian Journal of Trauma, Resuscitation and Emergency Medicine, 27, p. 88. Available at: https://doi.org/10.1186/s13049-019-0662-y

Hassankhani, H., Haririan, H., Porter, J.E., Heaston, S. (2018). Cultural aspects of death notification following cardiopulmonary resuscitation. *Journal of Advanced Nursing*, 74(7), pp. 1564–1572.

Heaston, S., Beckstrand, R.L., Bond, A.E., Palmer, S.P. (2006). Emergency nurses' perceptions of obstacles and supportive behaviors in end-of-life care. *Journal of Emergency Nursing*, 32(6), pp. 477–485.

Hobgood, C., Mathew, D., Woodyard, D.J., Shofer, F.S., Brice, J.H. (2013). Death in the field: Teaching paramedics to deliver effective death notifications using the educational intervention "GRIEV_ING". *Prehospital Emergency Care*, 17(4), pp. 501–510.

Jackson, V.A., Sullivan, A.M., Gadmer, N.M., Seltzer, D., Mitchell, A.M., Lakoma, M.D., Arnold, R.M., Block, S.D. (2005). "It was haunting…": Physicians' descriptions of emotionally powerful patient deaths. *Academic Medicine*, 80(7), pp. 648–656.

Králová, J. (2015). What is social death? *Contemporary Social Science*, 10(3), pp. 235–248.

Linklater, G.T. (2010). Educational needs of foundation doctors caring for dying patients. *Journal of the Royal College of Physicians Edinburgh*, 40(1), pp. 13–18.

Lock, M. (2002). *Twice dead: Organ transplants and the reinvention of death*. Berkeley: University of California Press.

Marco, C.A., Wetzel, L.R. (2012). Communication with survivors of motor vehicle crashes. *Emergency Medical Journal*, 29, pp. 626–629.

McClement, S.E., Fallis, W.M., Pereira, A. (2009). Family presence during resuscitation: Canadian critical care nurses' perspectives. *Journal of Nursing Scholarship*, 41(3), pp. 233–240.

Meier, D.E., Back, A.L., Morrison, R.S. (2001). The inner life of physicians and care of the seriously ill. *JAMA: The Journal of the American Medical Association*, 286(23), pp. 3007–3014.

Mills, L.D., Mills, T.J. (2005). Symptoms of post-traumatic stress disorder among emergency medicine residents. *Journal of Emergency Medicine*, 28(1), pp. 1–4.

Mitchell, J.T. (2008). A short guide to giving bad news. *International Journal of Emergency Mental Health*, 10(3), pp. 197–202.

Naik, S.B. (2013). Death in the hospital: Breaking the bad news to the bereaved family. *Indian Journal of Critical Care Medicine*, 17(3), pp. 178–181.

Neimeyer, R.A., Prigerson, H.G., Davies, B. (2002). Mourning and meaning. *American Behavioural Scientist*, 46(2), pp. 235–251.

Ombres, R., Montemorano, L., Becker, D. (2017). Death notification: Someone needs to call the family. *Journal of Palliative Medicine*, 20(6), pp. 672–675.

Parris, R.J. (2011). Initial management of bereaved relatives following trauma. *Trauma*, 14(2), pp. 139–155.

Redinbaugh, E.M., Sullivan, A.M., Block, S.D., Gadmer, N.M., Lakoma, M., Mitchell, A.M., Seltzer, D., Wolford, J., Arnold, R.M. (2003). Doctors' emotional reactions to recent death of a patient: Cross sectional study of hospital doctors. *British Medical Journal*, 327(7408), p. 185.

Roe, E. (2012). Practical strategies for death notification in the emergency department. *Journal of Emergency Nursing*, 38(2), pp. 130–134.

Smith, T.L., Walz, B.J., Smith, R.L. (1999). A death education curriculum for emergency physicians, paramedics, and other emergency personnel. *Prehospital Emergency Care*, 3(1), pp. 37–41.

Strote, J., Schroeder, E., Lemos, J., Paganelli, R., Solberg, J., Range Hutson, H.(2011). Academic emergency physicians' experiences with patient death. *Academic Emergency Medicine*, 18(3), pp. 255–260.

Stewart, A.E. (1999). Complicated bereavement and posttraumatic stress disorder following fatal car crashes: Recommendations for death notification. *Death Studies*, 23(4), pp. 289–321.

Sudnow, D. (1967). *Passing on*. Hoboken, NJ: Prentice-Hall.

Timmermans, S. (1998). Social death as self-fulfilling prophecy: David Sudnow's passing on revisited. *The Sociological Quarterly*, 39(3), pp. 453–472.

Tuffrey-Wijne, I., Rose, T. (2017). Investigating the factors that affect the communication of death-related bad news to people with intellectual disabilities by staff in residential and supported living services: an interview study. *Journal of Intellectual Disability Research*, 61(8), pp. 727–736.

Whippen, D.A., Canellos, G.P. (1991). Burnout syndrome in the practice of oncology: Results of a random survey of 1,000 oncologists. *Journal of Clinical Oncology*, 9(10), pp. 1916–1920.

Chapter 6

Making sense of death in the Emergency Department

Death has a significance beyond the physical realm, as established in the earlier chapters, as such, following an in-depth exploration of how this phenomenon is experienced, this chapter will seek to explore healthcare professional's (HCP) interpretation of death, beyond its biological or clinical description. Views of participants in my study ranged from 'mystifying death' or seeing death as a loss or separation, to being pragmatic, perhaps considering death as being 'part of the job'. The impact that values and norms have in the 'sense-making exercise' when HCPs are experiencing death often lead to labelling the phenomenon as being 'unfair', 'good', or 'out of norm'. This chapter will also explore the ethical and moral challenges and dilemmas HCPs will face, when dealing with death, and how clinical priorities can be shaped by their personal values and norms. Finally, the role of faith and spiritual beliefs will be discussed, and how spirituality often can affect the way HCPs cope with the experience of death in the Emergency Department (ED). We will examine how these views can provide comfort and protection against the negative impact of these experiences and in what way are able to shape the provision of care.

The meaning behind death

Understanding the study participants' values started by exploring what death itself meant to them and how they defined it. Some talked about death as a complex phenomenon and being difficult to describe. Erica, one of the nurses, for example, had no personal experience with death in the family, prior of starting to work in the ED, and described her sense-making of death, as being mystified by it.

> I thought of my two experiences in the ED, I had no previous experience with death, no family members, no friends - touch wood - I had no real concept of it, it was just black and white, you die, that's it. I could imagine it must be horrific, but I didn't really know what it be like. That was something, even as a student, I was always very worried happening, while I was a nurse, as I have no experience of what is like for someone to die.
>
> (Erica, Nurse)

DOI: 10.4324/9781032660912-6

More experienced members of staff, in a senior role, also referred to death as something which has no clear description. Christine reflected on death suggesting that the more she learned about it, the less she knows about it. Giving death a generalised definition is almost impossible as it is an individual experience.

> The obvious description of death is a human passing away and departing to heaven or whatever, depending, if they have a religion or not. There are different ways in which people die, different environments in which people die, some people react differently to death, family, friends, colleagues. So, I don't really think there's a clear description in my opinion, but people could have a different understanding of it.
>
> (Christine, Senior Sister)

For some participants death represented nothing more than a pragmatic reality, simply ceasing to exist. Participants sharing this approach viewed death as a cessation of biological processes and activities of the body, a natural, scientific state. Often participants when expressing their views on death expressed their spiritual 'standpoint' at the same time. Those defining death purely as a biological process referred often to themselves as 'atheists' or as someone who doesn't share any religious views.

> So, death for me means not existing anymore. So that means to me that your heart is not beating, you are not breathing, and you have no brain activity. That's what death means to me, it's an endpoint. I don't have religious beliefs, I don't believe in an afterlife, I'm an atheist, so when you die that's it.
>
> (Robert, Advanced Clinical Practitioner)

> But death for me is quite a scientific thing, something happened, and this person is not alive anymore. As I said I don't have religious beliefs, so I don't believe in afterlife.
>
> (Isaac, Charge Nurse)

> I think death is a natural part of life. For me it's just a natural thing that will happen to all of us. It's a natural end to a life. Obviously, this can be untimely, but for me I think talking about it in a general way it's an inevitable thing, just a natural part, like happiness and sadness and that is just a natural thing associated with life.
>
> (William, Registrar)

Similarly, those participants who were seeing death as more than a natural process, part of something greater than the end of biological existence, identified themselves predominantly as holding Christian beliefs. Death in their view is described as a 'separation', or 'being with God'. Death for some participants even meant the beginning of a new life.

> Death for me is when a person is no longer alive in a physical sense. Yet from my perspective as a Christian, it is more to us than just a physical body. So, death is a separation I guess between the physical body and the essence of a person, that being which is no longer present in a physical body. And you can tell, you know, when somebody dies that they are no longer there and there is something that is gone and no longer there.
>
> (Adam, Registrar)

> I think death is something … losing someone, but in a way as well it's the time to be with God, and I think it's very important when a person is dying to give them peace before dying. I think it's a new life, being with God.
>
> (Zoe, Senior Sister)

Other participants, who did not identify themselves as being religious or upholding a faith, still associated death with spirituality, referring to it as a departure to a 'better place', where pain ceased to exist. Charlie, for example, highlights that experiencing death regularly developed the need to find a meaning for this phenomenon.

> Interviewer: What does death mean to you personally?
>
> Participant: This is a very good question, it's one that I often ask myself a lot of the time. Especially when we deal with it so frequently. The whole honest answer, I wouldn't say I'm religious, I appreciate religious values, and I would say I am spiritual in a sense, I'd like to think it's someone going to a better place without suffering, without pain and they are going to be with their loved ones.
>
> (Charlie, Healthcare Assistant)

While some participants talked about being raised in a Christian family and still sharing these values as adults, Rachel, who was similarly born in such a family, does not share these values and while she respects them, they don't impact on her view or definition about death.

> I guess from maybe a personal point of view, my close and extended family are very Christian, and so what death means to them and the way I was brought up is that when people die, some people go to hell and some people go to heaven. That is something that I've been brought up but not necessarily believe.
>
> (Rachel, Advanced Clinical Practitioner)

One of the frequent interpretations of death given by many participants was that it is a component of their everyday job in the ED. This suggests that death, in this line of work, is perceived as something not 'out of the ordinary', something to be expected, even if the circumstances of the death are unexpected. Seeing death as 'normal' could lead to the development of an emotional numbness, as described by some participants, 'not feeling anything' when someone dies. This view could also contribute to the development of an invisible protection against the negative influence of these experiences.

> From a work point of view, I see it as part of the job, something that we expect to see, and I realize when we have people coming through our department and haven't experienced that and can have a very different emotional response to it. But I see it as a fundamental part of what we do.
>
> (Andrew, Consultant)

> I often see horrific things, but I say that's the job.
>
> (Julie, Healthcare Assistant)

> It has become so, normal for me as a nurse and probably as an ED nurse, that it's part of the job.
>
> (Christine, Senior Sister)

Participants, sometimes following prompting for a more diverse description in the interview, often described death as an event that has wider implications psychologically, emotionally, and socially. The euphemism 'loss', used for death, suggests a void that a person leaves behind in their family, job, society, and the world. Death was often viewed as being very difficult for the grieving family with complex ramifications in all areas of life.

> I think death has a massive impact, emotionally is difficult for everyone losing a loved one, a person who's had a life, for I don't know how many years, has made an impact on society, on the world in some way and they are no longer there, leaving their family, friends, job …
>
> (Margaret, Sister)

> Death to me is something that is exceptionally sad and it's life-changing for the people that are left behind. I always wondered that the actual act of dying is easy, it's the ramifications of that is the hard part.
>
> (David, Senior Charge Nurse)

The impact of individual values and norms

Whenever participants referred to death using an adjective, such as 'normal', 'good', 'common', or 'natural' they associated their own values and norms with that definition. Most participants associated the death of an elderly person as 'normal', while the death of a child was described differently. When death occurred due to 'natural' causes that was labelled as 'good' or 'normal'. Conversely, when death occurred unexpectedly, at a young age, for example, not allowing for that person to mature, death was seen as out of the norm.

> So, death at old age is a normal thing, that's a normal life thing. It's a common thing, we all die at the end of our life, depending on what life path we've had.

> When older people die just of natural things, that is a good place to be, I think. It's not always necessarily a bad thing. I think when death is sudden, unexpected, it's a shock, especially when a child dies. Suddenly and unexpectedly, I would say that is a big shock because that is not a natural life path, like a young person it should grow old, if that make sense.
>
> (Mary, Sister)

One of the frequent classifications that reflects personal values and norms associated with death were the notions of 'good' and 'bad' deaths. A 'good death' is associated with dignity, comfort, not being exposed to pain and suffering, not having ongoing futile and unnecessary treatments, and preferably dying with the family members present, whenever possible, in a familiar environment.

> I want people to have a good death. I think for me that means hopefully pain-free, hopefully free of unnecessary interventions; I prefer it if they could die at home. And I think recently we have managed to do that a few times … which is being good, I guess.
>
> (Robert, Advanced Clinical Practitioner)

Unlike ward-based settings, where deterioration is often gradual and relationships with patients can develop over time, the ED presents a rapid, often a seemingly chaotic environment, in which death may occur suddenly. This contrast illustrates the need for adaptability, emotional resilience, and acute clinical judgement. John, one of the interviewed junior doctors, also reveals how personal loss can shape professional values, fostering empathy and a deep commitment to quality care at the end of life.

> So, I lost my dad when I was 19, due to pancreatic cancer, so care for the end-of-life patient is really important to me. You can't do it again if you get it wrong. In the ED there is a very different timescale of death versus the wards where you look after a patient for weeks and deteriorate in time. In the ED people come to you and arrest, so it's a very different kind of tempo of death experience.
>
> (John, Junior Doctor)

Stopping active treatment of a patient was an aspect described by some participants as the most challenging part of the death and dying experience. Described often as a 'difficult balance' between clinical judgement, family wishes, and patient's interest, these decisions were infused by the professional, institutional, and personal values of the individual. Often families will require from HCPs working in the ED to initiate treatments that will not change the outcome, only will prolong the dying process, potentially undermining the possibility of a dignified death. Families, however, may use these opportunities to cling to any final hopes of recovery and delay saying goodbye to their loved ones.

> So, it wasn't unexpected just a really challenging process to bring them to the same page where we were. I wouldn't say we ED doctors are blunt, but we are

> very honest about a patient's condition, but the family was not on the same page at all. There was a lot of talking about what we can and can't do, and actually to come in say goodbye to him. He was with us for 12 hours in the Resus, and we didn't feel that there is anything else we could do to alter the course.
>
> (Andrew, Consultant)

Experiencing death in the family, and being influenced by personal values, can have an impact on how someone defines death, and how that reflects in their clinical practice. Zoe moved to the UK from the Southeast Asian region, and she was working in the ED when her grandparents died. She was unable to travel home and see them while they were still alive. She talked about, how she would have wanted to hold their hands, and offer them peace in their last moments, as that felt 'the right thing to do'. This event influenced her definition of a dignified and 'good death'. Therefore, in her practice, whenever she deals with dying patients, she endeavours to offer them opportunities to spend time with their family, even at the expense of delaying the transfer of the patient to the operating theatre.

> If the family is here, I try to make sure, they see them before they go to the theatre, as you don't know if they are going to make it, so that is really important for me. I would argue even with the doctor if they don't want to, just even a minute on the corridor, just to hold their hand. It's important to see them, because you can never know if they are going to make it in the theatre.
>
> (Zoe, Senior Sister)

Nicholas describes his experience with the family of a patient who died a very traumatic death, in relation to a complex moral dilemma. As the family was asking about the circumstances of death, Nicholas knew he didn't want to lie; however, he also does not want to expose the family to unnecessary suffering either. His immediate reaction to this complex situation was wanting to avoid it.

> I remember how I had a conversation with the family afterwards as well. I have been asked really hard questions by the family about what happened, and I had to go to the post-mortem. I remember they've asked me a really hard question: 'Was it quick?' … Wow … Ahhh … You didn't want to lie to them but how to say the whole truth about this guy chocking on his own vomit? I certainly wanted to run from that situation.
>
> (Nicholas, Consultant)

Trying to find a meaning to 'justify' the death of a child is sometimes part of the acceptance process of that death. Sometimes this meaning is found in the physical characteristics of a child, being more vulnerable and fragile compared to an adult. Another factor that makes the death of a child difficult is the thought of how parents are going to cope with this event, as it goes against the social norm of children dying before their parents.

> I think if an adult would have been hit by a motorcycle, they would have survived, and I think I wouldn't felt so bad, because the outcome would have been different. They would have probably gone for a surgery, but they would have survived.
>
> (Julie, Healthcare Assistant)

> With the kids it's always the thought of the impact on the parents and just knowing that two hours just changes everything forever for them. I think before being a parent I was cognisant of that.
>
> (Robert, Advanced Clinical Practitioner)

A child's death was often linked by the study participants to a moral duty and an ethical responsibility, that somehow, something needs to be done to save that life. Other times the death of a child left a feeling of void and emptiness in participants, often avoiding facing their own feelings after the event.

> I found it really hard, I have never been involved in a case that took so long for a child to end up dying. What I found really hard, is what to do next, once the case is finished. Everyone steps down, the team disperses, the parents are there with the child and what do you do now? I've been doing this all morning and what I did was, I had a drink, and I went to see another patient. Which I think it was the worst thing I could have done …
>
> (Andrew, Consultant)

Professional or institutional values reflect in many of the answers provided by the study participants, for example, when they refer to death and dying, as something that "goes against everything you want to do as a doctor or a nurse". Conversations with patients and family members, about death and dying, could raise several ethical and moral dilemmas. Telling a patient that they are actively dying or telling the family the truth about the real details of a traumatic death often put participants in an uncomfortable position, where their decision how to pursue that situation was guided by their ethical and moral standards.

> I find it actually quite hard telling someone that they are dying because it goes against everything you want to do as a doctor or nurse, trying to make them better, and part of me feels like, do you want them to know that, but then it's not your right to deprive them that information, because they need to know that really, but I find that quite hard to have that conversation.
>
> (Adam, Registrar)

Life-saving interventions in the ED are often continued, despite knowing it's futile, for the sake of the family being present, or in some cases for the sake of clinical staff. When the condition of a patient reaches a point, where every further treatment or intervention proves to be unsuccessful, the decision to continue a resuscitation is not based on clinical judgement, but moral principles, especially when family members are also present. As one of the participants described it, at that point the focus of the care shifts from the patient to the family. The decision to carry on with a procedure or treatment is to offer comfort and peace of mind for family members, knowing that the clinical team has done everything in their power to save the patient's life.

> And the hardest part is when you bring that family in and resuscitate that child even though you know it's futile and just doing compressions for the mum to see and then stop. That is probably the hardest thing.
>
> (Mary, Sister)

> Everyone came to realize that this child is too sick to move, but you continue resuscitation as the parents were there. Yet this case turned into a focusing our care on to them. He was probably four hours with us before we've stopped resuscitation.
>
> (Andrew, Consultant)

> I think making decisions to stop, if anything, I think we give people more time than medically we probably need to.
>
> (Adam, Registrar)

Ethical dilemmas surrounding death and dying can arise in various forms in the ED. William, one of the doctors interviewed, describes two different experiences with two different outcomes. In the first he describes a case where, despite all efforts of the team, the decision was to stop all active treatments for a patient and let him slowly die. He was expected to see other patients and walking away from that dying patient made him feel guilty. In the other similar case, he argues that while it is sad that he as a doctor can't spend more time with a dying patient, yet in the reality of the ED it's 'unfair' towards the other patients, to delay their treatment.

> Looking back, I feel guilty about this, when I look back to that situation. Because I walked away, I almost feel that my actions were almost inhumane, because I walked away from this man who was taking his last breath, and I carried on with my life.
>
> (William, Registrar)

> I know it's a very difficult ethical situation, but it wouldn't be right for me when a patient needs that loving support, yet it wouldn't be fair if I am one of the 2 registrars on a night shift to stay with this patient for the next hour. It is not feasible in reality. It is not possible, so I can't do that basically.
>
> (William, Registrar)

The role of faith and spiritual beliefs

Participants of my study often expressed their views about death, as being portrayed in the Western culture, as an event surrounded by sadness. Some participants talked about the need to concentrate on the positives of a human life and re-focus from the sadness of the moment. For many participants, the belief that the deceased patient is going to a 'better place', a place without pain, suggests that this offers them mechanisms for coping with death. A protection against experiencing a range of negative emotions associated with grieving and a comfort that helps with coping.

> I would say I am more and more open to perspectives of how people are seeing death. I am fascinated how historically we used to celebrate people dying, you know going to a better place. Especially in other cultures it's a celebration of life … we should look at the positives and I think to have that you've got to believe that wherever they are going it's a better place, where they are not in pain.
>
> (Charlie, Healthcare Assistant)

Participants who defined themselves as having faith or religious beliefs often talked about the influence of their spirituality on their experience with death. Julie, who works mostly with children, defined her faith as a support in maintaining a positive, optimistic view and remaining empathetic. Her spirituality played an important role in not developing avoidance as a coping mechanism. However, her values influenced her views on accepting some deaths as being 'normal', while others were seen as out of norm.

> Do you think without this faith your experience would be very much different?
>
> Participant: Yes. Probably I would be either more pessimistic or I couldn't be bothered, saying that it's just a life there are many more in the world. When elderly come in, then die, my 'work self' says that they had a good life, and it's normal that they died at that age. But when a 20-year-old comes in and dies, my 'Catholic self' says, that's not fair, that's not God's plan.
>
> (Julie, Healthcare Assistant)

When death occurred outside of the hierarchy of values a participant was holding, often faith and personal values were put to test and their validity questioned, when a death apparently was meaningless for participants. Yet, the same values contributed to them finding comfort and meaning.

> I didn't understand how a beautiful girl who didn't do anything wrong in her life could lost her life so tragically … And as a Catholic you go against your religion, asking 'Why are you doing this?' Like adults, old people fair enough take them; but children? And you do question your faith sometimes, saying this isn't fair. But it's all in His hand.
>
> (Julie, Healthcare Assistant)

Praying as an act of faith was often used by some participants, as a method of coping and processing difficult, traumatic situations, when experiencing the death of their patients. Prayer was not only defined as an act to restore personal confidence, but it was also used as part of the holistic care provided to the grieving family.

> And sometimes I do crossover, and I am standing next to a bed, and I am praying quietly, because that's my belief, to ask for help and strength for myself, because I see horrific things.
>
> (Julie, Healthcare Assistant)

> When they come to the viewing room, I pray for them, silently … I just stay there and pray for them. I do. I don't know what religion they are, but I pray for them.
>
> (Zoe, Senior Sister)

Personal values were reflected in how HCPs interpreted the death of children, often associated with a personal failure. While the death of an adult is often seen as 'acceptable', a child is seen as someone who needs protection, and if death occurs in the ED, that could be interpreted as the inability to fulfil the requirements of the clinical role.

> With situations involving children I am much more sensitive. I don't like the fact that a child must come to the Resus Room for whatever reason. I'm supposed to protect them. If I can't protect them, then I am not good for this. This is the way I see things. This is what I believe.
>
> (Annabelle, Healthcare Assistant)

Discussion: making sense of death in the Emergency Department

In my empirical study, HCPs described their personal views and understanding of the meaning of death in multiple ways. Some described it as something difficult to comprehend, or purely as the end of biological processes in the human body, while others have associated death with fundamental changes in the psychological, emotional, social, and spiritual dimension of all those involved in the process. Understanding death is deeply rooted into the philosophical investigation of two questions. The first question is conceptual or ontological, 'What is human death?' and the second questions is epistemological, 'How can someone determine that it has occurred?' (Green and Wikler, 1980; Halevy and Brody, 1993; Veatch, 2019). However, philosophical debate about death is not limited to these two questions, as a deeper understanding, requires an exploration of how the death of a human being is related or connected to other living beings, and if death reaches beyond biology, along what wider basis should be defined? (Bagheri, 2007).

The concept of death in the Classical Antiquity was influenced by the Greek medicine, especially by the work of Hippocrates, describing the body as a system, claiming that death occurs when the balance of the four humours is lost (Nutton, 2012). Hippocrates' humoral theory, later adapted by Galen, states that the imbalance of the four main bodily fluids (humours): blood, phlegm, yellow bile, and black bile are responsible for illness and ultimately for death (Bhikha and Glynn, 2017). This theory influenced not just medicine but also psychology, philosophy, and literature, and persisted until the 17th century, when modern anatomy and physiology began to replace it. Later, in the 18th–19th century, following the rise of autopsy and pathology, and the discovery of the stethoscope, significantly improving the detection of a heartbeat, death was considered the irreversible cessation of cardiopulmonary and respiratory function, and as such an irreversible cessation of functioning of the organism as a whole (Becker, 1975). The 20th century witnesses the introduction of electroencephalogram (EEG) to detect brain activity and neurologists create an early definition of brain-death, while technological advancements in organ donation, at the dawn of the 21st century, drive the need for a precise death criterion, yet in the same time advanced imaging technologies, such as CT (computed tomography) and MRI (magnetic resonance imaging), blur the lines between life and death even more. Traditionally, a patient who suffered a severe injury of the brain and brainstem resulted in a respiratory failure leading to cardiac arrest, which in return if it was prolonged, led to an irreversible loss of brain function (Veatch, 1976). The 'whole brain' approach defines human death as being an irreversible cessation of functioning of the entire brain, including the brainstem, while previously a 'brain-dead' patient was considered alive, if respiration (even assisted) still occurred (Cranford, 1995; Bernat, 2006). A progressive alternative offered is the 'higher brain' approach, which defines human death as being an irreversible cessation of the capacity for consciousness (McMahan, 2002). The term 'consciousness' refers to a state, in which patients can sustain a

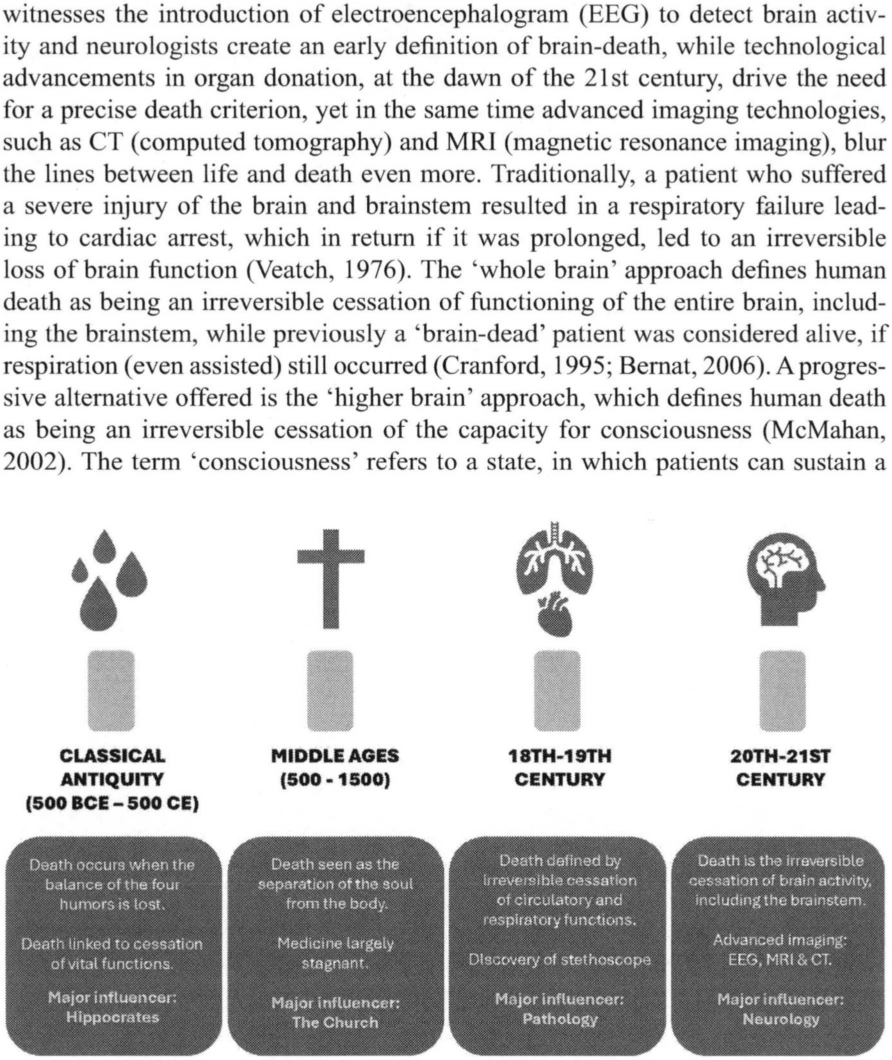

Figure 6.1 Major concepts of biological death over history.

functioning neurological system, including those in a reversible coma, being considered to be still alive (Baker, 2000). The major milestones in defining biological death throughout history are presented in Figure 6.1.

This idea is rooted in the interpretation that a person has an 'essence', a capacity for 'consciousness', without which we wouldn't exist (DeGrazia, 1999). This approach is also linked to the idea of loss of personal identity and the idea that death is also a moral question, in a sense that certain behaviours are appropriate, while others are not, such as grieving, organ donation, or burial (DeGrazia, 2005; Green and Wikler, 1980). Some modern alternatives define death as a process, not as a determinate event, arguing that organisms can't fully belong to either sets of existence, life or death, because the boundary between them is not perfectly sharp (Halevy and Brody, 1993; Youngner et al., 1999). Traditional interpretation of death focused on the physical aspects, while often overlooking the spiritual dimension. Yet, at the end of their lives, patients often wish to re-examine their beliefs, to reiterate spiritual values, to have closure and die peacefully, so the implications of death in the spiritual realm require recognition (Choundry et al., 2018). Participants of my study have also given various interpretations to death, most of them acknowledging that a generalised definition is almost impossible to be given, death being an individual experience, sometimes even difficult to conceptualise.

The study of Cevik and Kav (2013) surveyed 300 Turkish nurses about their attitudes and experiences towards death and caring for the dying patients. Forty-five percent of the nurses reflected on their religious views greatly affecting their attitude towards death and the dying patient. Less fear and avoidance of death was noted in the nurses who defined themselves as having strong religious beliefs, in comparison to the nurses who didn't (Cevik and Kav, 2013). Although the findings of a Korean study that surveyed 230 nurses concluded that a better performance in end-of-life care is mostly dependant on the positive perceptions of death and attitude towards end-of-life care itself. These findings are consistent with the results of my study, placing the positive attitude towards death ahead of religious beliefs, when personal views impact the care provided for the dying patient and their families. The role of faith and religious beliefs in making sense, coping with death, or offering holistic support for families was also supported by my study.

Situations surrounding the death and dying, which were challenging the moral integrity of the participants of my study, were frequently reported. Ethical and moral dilemmas surrounding death were primary elements of the death experiences in my study, including labelling death, such as 'good', 'normal', or 'unfair', taking moral decisions to stop active treatment or to prolong resuscitation, or quite the opposite, carrying on with a life-saving procedure. Other studies also suggest that emergency clinicians repeatedly reported a conflict arising from the life-saving ethos characteristic to the ED and providing end-of-life care in the same environment (Grudzen et al., 2012a, b; Murphy, 2008). A Dutch study conducted among physicians of all specialities found that 62% of them agreed that receiving futile and invasive investigations or treatments for patients near death is very common, mainly because preserving and lengthening life is the default medical approach (Visser, 2012). These findings are consistent with an Australian study, in which 65% of the surveyed physicians believed that many patients nearing their end-of-life, receive medical treatment when presenting to the ED, which is unlikely to benefit them and as such, represents a barrier in providing adequate care (Marck et al., 2014). Participants of my study agreed that stopping active treatments that proved to be futile is a difficult balance between clinical judgement and family wishes, clinicians trying to offer a dignified death to their patients, while families cling to their final hopes in saving their relative.

Omoya et al. (2022) conducted a study in Australia, interviewing seven emergency doctors and nine emergency nurses, while reached to the conclusion that determining if a treatment should be considered futile, not only clinical considerations, but in each individual case, ethical aspects should also be weighed. Another study, interviewing 16 Spanish emergency nurses, concluded that ethical dilemmas in the ED, surrounding palliative patients, arise from a conflict between doctors, who will sometimes consider only the medical aspect to pursue a solution, and nurses, who will make an effort to be advocates for their patients' best interest, feeling often helpless (Jimenez-Herrera and Axelsson, 2015). Participants in this study sometimes referred to death, as something that happens even before the biological cessation of life, when the patient stops interacting, when they stop being the person they were before and when an emotional disconnect surfaces.

My empirical study described certain ethical dilemmas when providing resuscitation for a child, with the parents and carers allowed to be present during a resuscitation attempt in the hospital. However, often there is a controversy surrounding this question. Those arguing for parents to be present during their child's resuscitation say that parents can have a better insight into reality and have a chance to say goodbye, in case the attempt is unsuccessful, helping them in the grieving process. Opposing to this idea, some parents, who lost their child under such circumstances, say that they wish not to remember seeing their child dying (Tsiligiri et al., 2010; Shaw et al., 2011). Those arguing for parents not to be present claim that they could interfere with clinical procedures, can affect staff's technical performance and stress level, and potentially undermine medical decision-making (Curley et al., 2012; Tripon et al., 2014). Decision to carry on with the resuscitation of a child when parents were present, even knowing that it's futile, was driven by the personal and professional values of HCPs interviewed in my study.

Participants of my study often expressed their affiliation to a particular faith, and how these spiritual values shaped their view about death and guided their clinical work. For almost all of the interviewed HCPs, the spiritual dimension of death had a great significance, even for those that didn't consider themselves as being religious. Miner-Williams (2006) argues that spirituality is an "integrative energy and the transcendent quest for meaning and happiness", which leads to health and the relief of sufferings. Spirituality represents more than religion, being rooted in the meaning of life, becoming more important when one experiences life crisis, such as being diagnosed with terminal illness or nearing end of life (Vermandere et al., 2012). The same idea is shared by Sulmasy (2009), who claims that spirituality is a broader concept, in which is compatible with all forms of religious beliefs, moreover even with the absence or rejection of faith. The relationship between HCPs working in the ED and patients at the end of their life should include spiritual care, based on the assessment of the patient's individual spiritual needs (Seccareccia and Brown, 2009). Many of the participants of my study explicitly expressed the absence of religious beliefs, yet still referred to spirituality as a 'guiding compass' in making sense of the death experience.

Some studies suggest that nurses have significantly more positive attitudes than doctors towards the importance of spiritual care, as historically, nursing has always incorporated this type of care, such as Florence Nightingale's initiative to introduce music in the environment to facilitate the healing process (Balboni et al., 2013; Phelps et al., 2012; Nightingale, 1860). As obstacles in providing spiritual care, ED staff highlights time pressures and the inability to discover and understand dying patient and their family's spiritual background (Balboni et al., 2014). There are conflicting views about supporting patients to observe their religious beliefs as part of the spiritual care. Staff participating in some studies argue that religion is something very personal to them and they would avoid bringing it up (Keall et al., 2014), while others argue that education on the differing views of various religions may help to accept patients' views better (Yingting et al., 2018). Involvement of chaplaincy service is viewed as useful in addressing patients and family members' needs of spiritual care (Puchalski et al., 2006). The need and significance to involve chaplaincy services in dealing with and supporting the grieving family, was often mentioned by the participants of my study as well. Spirituality and faith played an important role in dealing with death for many of the participants of my study, shaping the way they interpret the meaning of death, while for others manifested in practices that supported them in coping with the death experience, but also aided the spiritual support they provided for the bereaved family.

Experiences in my study are supported by the findings of Wu and Volker (2009), who argues that nurses who consider religious beliefs important building blocks of their personhood tend to deal with traumatic events, such as the sudden or unexpected death of their patient, by adopting a more purposeful and positive approach. Ho et al. (2022) also suggest that the death and dying experiences could strengthen the faith and spirituality of those nurses who hold religious beliefs. Ntantana et al. (2017) surveyed 149 intensive care doctors and 320 intensive care nurses in Greece to explore the impact of HCPs' personality and religious beliefs on the decisions to forego life-sustaining treatments. The study found that the more religious a HCP was, the more reluctant it appeared to withdraw life-sustaining mechanical ventilation, considered by many a 'passive euthanasia'. A link between religious views and negative attitudes towards withdrawal of active therapy was also found by another study among Iranian students of Muslim faith (Aghababaei and Wasserman, 2013). On the contrary, religious faith had predominantly positive influence on the participants of my study, sometimes being 'tested' by certain death experiences, but predominantly offering support in having a positive attitude, coping, and provide holistic care.

Reference list

Aghababaei, N., Wasserman, J.A. (2013). Attitude toward euthanasia scale: Psychometric properties and relations with religious orientation, personality and life satisfaction. *American Journal of Hospice and Palliative Medicine*, 30(8), pp. 781–785.

Bagheri, A. (2007). Individual choice in the definition of death. *Journal of Medical Ethics*, 33(3), pp. 146–149.

Baker, L.R. (2000). *Persons and bodies*. Cambridge: Cambridge University Press.

Balboni, M.J., Sullivan, A., Amobi, A., Phelps, A.C., Gorman, D.P., Zollfrank, A., Peteet, J.R., Prigerson, H.G., Balboni, T.A. (2013). Why is spiritual care infrequent at the end of life? Spiritual care perceptions among patients, nurses, and physicians and the role of training. *Journal of Clinical Oncology*, 31(4), pp. 461–467.

Balboni, M.J., Sullivan, A., Enzinger, A.C., Epstein-Peterson, Z.D., Tseng, Y.D., Mitchell, C., Niska, J., Zollfrank, A., VanderWeele, T.J., Balboni, T.A. (2014). Nurse and physician barriers to spiritual care provision at the end of life. *Journal of Pain Symptom Management*, 48(3), pp. 400–410.

Becker, L. (1975). Human being: The boundaries of the concept. *Philosophy and Public Affairs*, 4(2), pp. 334–359.

Bernat, J. (2006). The whole-brain concept of death remains optimum public policy. *Journal of Law, Medicine & Ethics*, 34(1), pp. 35–43.

Bhikha, R., Glynn, J. (2017). The theory of humours revisited. *International Journal of Development Research*, 7(9), pp.15029–15034.

Cevik, B., Kav, S. (2013). Attitudes and experiences of nurses toward death and caring for dying patients in Turkey. *Cancer Nursing*, 36(6), pp. 58–65.

Choundry, M., Latif, A., Warburton, K.G. (2018). An overview of the spiritual importances of end-of-life care among the five major faiths of the United Kingdom. *Clinical Medicine*, 18(1), pp. 23–31.

Cranford, R. (1995). Criteria for death, in W. Reich (ed.), *Encyclopedia of bioethics* (2nd Edition). New York: Macmillan, pp. 529–534.

Curley, M.A., Meyer, E.C., Scoppettuolo, L.A., McGann, E.A., Trainor, B.P., Rachwal, C.M., Hickey, P.A. (2012). Parent presence during invasive procedures and resuscitation: Evaluating a clinical practice change. *American Journal of Respiratory Critical Care Medicine*, 186(11), pp. 1133–1139.

DeGrazia, D. (1999). Persons, organisms, and death: A philosophical critique of the higher-brain approach. *Southern Journal of Philosophy*, 37(3), pp. 419–40.

DeGrazia, D. (2005). *Human identity and bioethics*. Cambridge: Cambridge University Press.

Green, M., Wikler, D. (1980). Brain death and personal identity. *Philosophy and Public Affairs*, 9(2), pp. 105–33.

Grudzen, C.R., Lynne, D.R., Hannah, M.M., Brandon, K., Joanna, M.O., Morrison, R.S. (2012a). Hospital administrators' views on barriers and opportunities to delivering palliative care in the Emergency Department. *Annals of Emergency Medicine*, 61(6), pp. 654–660.

Grudzen, C.R., Richardson, L.D., Susan, S.H., Joanna, M.O., Christine, W., Morrison, R.S. (2012b). Does palliative care have a future in the Emergency Department? Discussions with attending emergency physicians. *Journal of Pain Symptom Management*, 43(1), pp. 1–9.

Halevy, A., Brody, B. (1993). Brain death: Reconciling definitions, criteria, and tests. *Annals of Internal Medicine*, 119(6), pp. 519–525.

Ho, C.Y., Lim, N., Ong, Y.T., Lee, A.S.I., Chiam, M., Gek, G.P.L., Sarraf-Yazdi, S., Mason, S., Krishna, L. (2022). The impact of death and dying on the personhood of senior nurses at the National Cancer Centre Singapore (NCCS): A qualitative study. *BMC Palliative Care*, 21, p. 83. Available at: https://doi.org/10.1186/s12904-022-00974-9

Jimenez-Herrera, M.F., Axelsson, C. (2015). Some ethical conflicts in emergency care. *Nursing Ethics*, 22(5), pp. 548–560.

Keall, R., Clayton, J.M., Butow, P. (2014). How do Australian palliative care nurses address existential and spiritual concerns? Facilitators, barriers and strategies. *Journal of Clinical Nursing*, 23(21–22), pp. 3197–3205.

Marck, C.H., Weil, J., Lane, H., Weiland, T.J., Philip, J., Boughey, M., Jelinek, G.A. (2014). Care of the dying cancer patient in the Emergency Department: Findings from a national survey of Australian Emergency Department clinicians. *Internal Medicine Journal*, 44(4), pp. 362–368.

McMahan, J. (2002). *The ethics of killings: Problems at the margins of life*. Oxford: Oxford University Press.

Miner-Williams, D. (2006). Putting a puzzle together: Making spirituality meaningful for nursing using an evolving theoretical framework. *Journal of Clinical Nursing*, 15(7), pp. 811–821.

Murphy, B.F. (2008). What has happened to clinical leadership in futile care discussions? *Medical Journal of Australia*, 188(7), pp. 418–419.

Nightingale, F. (1860). *Notes on nursing: What is it, and what it is not*. New York: D. Appleton and Company.

Ntantana, A., Matamis, D., Savvidou, S., Marmanidou, K., Giannakou, M., Gouva, M., Nakos, G., Koulouras, V. (2017). The impact of healthcare professionals' personality and religious beliefs on the decisions to forego life sustaining treatments: An observational, multicentre, cross-sectional study in Greek intensive care units. *BMJ Open*, 7(7), p. e013916.

Nutton, V. (2012). *Ancient medicine* (2nd Edition). London: Routledge.

Omoya, O., De Bellis, A., Breaden, K. (2022). Death, dying, and end-of-life care provision by doctors and nurses in the Emergency Department. *Journal of Hospice & Palliative Nursing*, 24(2), pp. 48–57.

Phelps, A.C., Lauderdale, K.E., Alcorn, S., Dillinger, J., Balboni, M.T., Wert, M.V., Vanderweele, T.J., Balboni, T.A. (2012). Addressing spirituality within the care of patients at the end of life: Perspectives of patients with advanced cancer, oncologists, and oncology nurses. *Journal of Clinical Oncology*, 30(20), pp. 25–38.

Puchalski, C.M., Lunsford, B., Harris, M.H., Miller, R.T. (2006). Interdisciplinary spiritual care for seriously ill and dying patients: A collaborative model. *Cancer Journal*, 12(5), pp. 398–416.

Seccareccia, D., Brown, J.B. (2009). Impact of spirituality on palliative care physicians: Personally and professionally. *Journal of Palliative Medicine*, 12(9), pp. 805–809.

Shaw, K., Ritchie, D., Adams, G. (2011). Does witnessing resuscitation help parents to come to the terms with the death of their child? A review of the literature. *Intensive and Critical Care Nursing*, 27(5), pp. 253–262.

Sulmasy, D.P. (2009). Spirituality, religion, and clinical care. *Chest Journal*, 135(6), pp. 1634–1642.

Tripon, C., Defossez, G., Ragot, S., Ghazali, A., BoureauVoultoury, A., Scépi, M., Oriot, D. (2014). Parental presence during cardiopulmonary resuscitation of children: The experience, opinions and moral positions of emergency teams in France. *Archives Disability Child*, 99(4), pp. 310–315.

Tsiligiri, M., Zioga, D., Orfanidou, M. (2010). Nursing care and parents contribution in the care of their children with hypospadias. *International Journal of Caring Sciences*, 3(3), pp. 106–109.

Yingting, Z., Yash Pal, R., Wai, T., Wilson, S., Lee, A., Ong, M., Hwaa, T.L. (2018). Spiritual perspectives of emergency medicine doctors and nurses in caring for end-of-life patients: A mixed-method study. *International Emergency Nursing*, 37, pp. 13–22.

Youngner, S., Arnold, R., Shapiro, R. (1999). *The definition of death: Contemporary controversies*. Baltimore, MD: Johns Hopkins University Press.

Veatch, R.M. (1976). *Death, dying, and the biological revolution*. New Haven, CT: Yale University Press.

Veatch, R.M. (2019). Controversies in defining death: A case for choice. *Theoretical Medicine and Bioethics*, 40(5), pp. 381–401.

Vermandere, M., Choi, Y.N., De Brabandere, H., Decouttere, R., De Meyere, E., Gheysens, E., Nickmans, B., Schoutteten, M., Seghers, L., Truijens, J., Vandenberghe, S., Van de Wiele, S., Oevelen, L.A.V., Aertgeerts, B. (2012). GPs' views concerning spirituality and the use of the FICA tool in palliative care in Flanders: A qualitative study. *British Journal of General Practice*, 62(603), pp. 718–725.

Visser, J. (2012). The doctor is in treatment mode. *Medical Contact*, 67, pp. 1326–1329.

Wu, H., Volker, D.L. (2009). Living with death and dying: The experience of Taiwanese hospice nurses. *Oncology Nursing Forum*, 36(5), pp. 578–584.

Chapter 7

The influence of death in the Emergency Department

Following an investigation into what makes some death experiences in the Emergency Department (ED) memorable and how healthcare professionals' (HCPs) values and norms influence this experience, this final chapter will investigate how this will impact their personal and professional life, underpinned by four major themes. 'Changed by death' describes how perspectives, behaviours, priorities, and personality of participants were affected by the death experience. 'The emotional labour of death' describes the wide range of emotions triggered by these experiences and the investment it requires to handle death and the dying, while 'Coping with death' explores the various ways participants choose to cope with them. Finally, 'Learning from death' describes what would be required to be better prepared for and how patient care or career perspectives are shaped by these death experiences.

Changed by death

Witnessing death in the ED is an experience that changed peoples' views about themselves and the world surrounding them, both professionally and personally. The death experience, according to the participants of my study, caused them to review their own behaviours, perspectives, priorities, and interactions, yet also to acknowledge the emotions associated with this experience. Some described the change they experienced in themselves as 'get used to it', 'become harsher', or as 'having no feelings at all'. This is often described as a gradual process that happens over the years and being changed by the experience of death in the ED was often perceived as almost inevitable. The only time some HCPs allow themselves to be affected emotionally is when they meet the relatives and are willing to offer a holistic support, making themselves 'vulnerable' again.

> After [several] years working in the ED, I have no feelings at all anymore seeing a dead person. There is nothing. It has become so, normal for me as a nurse and probably as an ED nurse, that it's part of the job. Normal in the ED, it happens, the only time I get upset probably is when I see the reactions of the family because that's when it really hits home.
>
> (Christine, Senior Sister)

DOI: 10.4324/9781032660912-7

> So, by the end of my foundation year I have seen a tremendous amount of death, and you learn to get used to it. I think it has impacted me in terms of my approach to death when it happens in the Emergency Department and certainly helped me to build a pile of experiences, for example with breaking the bad news, or select the right answers to people.
>
> (Nicholas, Consultant)

Experiencing death regularly influenced HCPs' approach to end-of-life care, clinical practice, and patient care, and improved their relationship with families, irrespective of their job role or professional rank. Changes were evident in the improvement of therapeutic communication skills, techniques in breaking the bad news to family members, spending more time with them instead of rushing to the next patient, and offering them a compassionate, empathetic support.

> Every case chip a little bit and steer your practice. Meeting relatives and breaking bad news overall is getting better. Finding the right phrases that convey the severity of the instance and the gravity of the news you are delivering in a compassionate manner is something that I am learning.
>
> (John, Junior Doctor)

> I think it made me empathize more with patients who are dying, or family members of patients who are dying, because I know exactly what it's like.
>
> (Christine, Senior Sister)

Erica, one of the nurses, described her experience of witnessing death, as something that changed her understanding about life and death.

> It sounds awful but it kind of makes you become more harsh and harder out to shout. Once I was finally over after the first one, I was proud of myself because I think I went through a low point of my life, finally being able to process something so horrific. It felt better and I've enjoyed my job again, and actually I felt quite good afterwards, around six months down the line. It definitely changed me as a person and made me aware of what life and death is.
>
> (Erica, Nurse)

Clinical practice and patient support were also changed in case of most participants often being rooted not only in the influence of the death experience, but also in their own values. Adam, one of the ED doctors, expressed his beliefs and Christian faith and how these affected his views on involving chaplaincy services in better supporting families during a time of grief. The expressions 'I always thought about' or 'I think it's really important' suggest that these changes in clinical practice are supported by the values and morals embedded within the death experience.

> But in terms of how death has affected me, I am always keen to have the family involved as soon as possible … One of the things that I always thought about

> and I had no chance to use it is things like the chaplaincy service, because I know they are available, they are there to support people … This is something that I would try to incorporate more into my practice.
>
> (Adam, Registrar)

Reviewing medical or clinical practices as a response to regularly being exposed to death was another significant element of the changes experienced by ED staff. Doctors talked about reviewing futile and unnecessary treatment, while focusing more on palliative medication and treatment to preserve dignity at the end of life. The changes observed in participants were gradual, as at the beginning of their career was mostly dominated by a 'getting them better at all costs' attitude, compared to a better understanding of end-of-life principles at a later, probably more mature stage of their career. The changes in practice, in the fast-paced environment of an ED, are also fuelled by the understanding that often there is only 'one chance' to provide the most appropriate care.

> You must know when to stop sometime, especially if they are an elderly patient and spending more time thinking about how to give them a dignified death. I think I have a more insight of that now than I had at the start of my career.
>
> (Adam, Registrar)

> I think the change comes from myself. Probably in terms of using palliative care medications and to allow the loved ones in even if it's two o'clock in the morning. I would let people come in and say goodbye, because as I said before, you can't take it back, you can't do it again.
>
> (John, Junior Doctor)

Witnessing death affected the HCPs in this study, both professionally and personally, changing their perspective, and views about the world and mortality. This experience allowed them often to reflect upon and acknowledge their own emotions, in contrast with carrying on, moving to the next case or patient.

> It certainly changes your perspective, your view of the world, it changes your view on mortality and death. Death has become very alien to the general population. Again, I speak in generalized terms, and you realize it's just the normal part of life.
>
> (William, Registrar)

> I am much more aware of the impact the cases will have on me. Whether it's being upset, frustration, anger, no matter what emotion is, it's important to have that.
>
> (Andrew, Consultant)

A change of priorities was also observed in participant's reflections on their death experiences, such as valuing time spent with their family and friends, valuing relationships, or taking every opportunity to express their gratitude. Some participants also reported on how these experiences made them realise how length of life can be relative and made them more inclined to prioritise, for example, travels and holidays.

> I think if you have a case where, or if you have a time when something bad happens at work, it makes you think, I just want to ring my dad. I just want to ring my mum and have a chat. Or you know, whatever it is, and I think it highlights how important family and friends are.
>
> (Rachel, Advanced Clinical Practitioner)

> You just learn to appreciate what you've got. And my kids, I'm just grateful that they are here. For my husband. You learn to appreciate things, I think.
>
> (Zoe, Senior Sister)

While putting on an 'armour' was perceived by HCPs as a detachment for their own wellbeing, allowing to 'maintain a distance', some staff consciously decided to become 'softer', to remove this protective barrier, and embrace the feelings associated with the death experience, making them more empathetic towards bereaved families.

> For some time, I was putting a shield on because you don't want to see what it is like to die. I have been involved in cases where multiple injured people are coming in, and you must put the shield on, to move on to the next patient. But I think since moving into paediatrics I have become a lot softer. I don't put that wall up anymore, because I don't have to. The more you do nursing, the more you feel you don't have to put that front up, you can be that person. When you speak with a bereaved family, and you start crying you know that the family will appreciate it.
>
> (Julie, Healthcare Assistant)

The emotional labour of death

Participants reflecting on their own feelings and emotional reactions to the death experience describe these feelings as ranging from sadness to fear. Participants often found this emotional state difficult to verbalise. Many suggested that these emotions evolved over time, being impacted by it more often at the beginning of their career, whilst later in their careers the experience became less distressing.

> There are so many emotions that you go through, like sadness, like the fear for that family, not knowing if they are going to cope … it's quite indescribable actually.
>
> (Mary, Sister)

> That was the first time I've seen a dead body, and I was very upset.
>
> (Christine, Senior Sister)

Sadness and fear, often associated with grieving, could be mixed with feelings of failure, a specific emotional state, many participants described as part of their death experience. The inability to save a life to change the course of events, despite all efforts, resources, and skills available, could potentially instigate self-blame in staff, questioning if all options were explored in the process.

> You grieve differently in your private life compared to someone you've never met. You still grieve but in a different way. I don't know if you can call it a professional grieve … You grieve for the family because you couldn't do all that you could do. We want to preserve and save life that's why we do our job. We want to make people better and fix them so they can walk out of the department. I guess it's a sense of grief and failure that we couldn't do that.
>
> (Mary, Sister)

Participants expressed that their emotions are not always visible, and even though some prefer to internalise these death-associated emotions, the intensity and the complexity remains the same. Staff suggested that the absence of these visible signs of grieving could be misinterpreted as someone being cold, distant, or less empathetic.

> Crying is the external representation of that emotion, but that does not mean if you are not crying you are not feeling sad. Or anger can be an external representation, but if you are quiet does not mean that you are not angry inside.
>
> (William, Registrar)

While ED is a fast-paced environment, with complex pressures on staff in dealing with a large number of patients over a certain period of time, participants described their time spent with a critically ill patient, as requiring an emotional investment. If that patient dies and clinical staff is required to pick the next case, they've found it difficult to make this sudden shift, as could jeopardise the quality of care and attention provided to that patient.

> Another aspect is the time you get involved with the case. Four hours with that child, 12 hours with the other case … it's an emotional investment there.
>
> (Andrew, Consultant)

> Just ask yourself the question: Am I the right person to do a procedure or give advice after I had such a difficult case? As a consultant you want people to look up to you and say, that they are calm and confident, they know what they are doing. But it's fine sometimes to take 5 minutes, have a drink and think.
>
> (Andrew, Consultant)

Emotional awareness is an integral part of dealing with the death experience, recognising, and acknowledging these emotions instead of bottling them up, or pretending that none of these experiences affect the individual. While emotional reactions can differ among staff, working as a team with the same patient, building a similar rapport, getting to know the family, will help sharing the emotional burden with the rest of the team as a measure of coping.

> Some people might feel different emotions, but in general if you are part of that core team, you make decisions as a team, so at the end the emotions you are feeling, would be similar. The core emotions would be similar.
>
> (William, Registrar)

> Be aware that things will affect us and it's okay to be affected. We shouldn't feel bad that we have these emotions, just understand how these emotions will affect you.
>
> (Andrew, Consultant)

Participants have expressed that embracing their own emotions helped them to have a more holistic approach in care and avoid an objectification of the patient. Participants of the study in general associated having emotions as an essential component or requirement for their profession.

> I think if I don't get affected anymore, I would leave my profession. I don't think it's the right job for you if you don't get affected anymore. It's part of being human, it's part of being a nurse to be able to empathize. If you wouldn't be able to empathize with the family or the patient than you are in the wrong profession.
>
> (Zoe, Senior Sister)

> I think it's good to have insight on things that affect us and how to look after each other and be aware that we are not robots, we are human beings, and we have emotions… We all need kindness, and we need to look after each other. I think when that's missing, people get too much focused on the patient and the outcomes.
>
> (Adam, Registrar)

Coping with death

Participants described various ways of coping with the death experience, and while these were different in each individual case, there were many similarities too. Some participants acknowledged that the way they cope with death is not healthy or beneficial to their wellbeing. One mechanism, some participants viewed, as being a least efficient way to cope, was by internalising emotions and not talking about these experiences, dealing with all associated emotions by themselves.

> I handle them in the worst way you could do it. I have insight that the way I handle them is not a healthy way and the way I handle them is lock them away and don't think about it. There are certain cases which are difficult and speaking with your team members is a good way to handle them. You realize that what you are feeling, everyone else is feeling the same.
>
> (William, Registrar)

> I think it's important to be able to talk about things and not bottle up emotions.
>
> (Rachel, Advanced Clinical Practitioner)

As methods of coping that proved to be unhealthy, participants mentioned alcohol consumption, smoking, or physical exercise taken to extremes. Some of the participants reported that they were aware that these do not offer a resolution, only a temporary numbing or distraction from these feelings.

> I think when I was younger, I drank a lot. I didn't had responsibility so kind of can do that, obviously that is not helpful. I went through a period a couple years ago, intense exercise, where I ran almost every day for two years. That doesn't work.
>
> (Robert, Advanced Clinical Practitioner)

Wearing the uniform as an 'armour' or a 'shield' was described by many participants as a way of protecting themselves from being deeply affected by the death experience. The same analogy re-surfaces in some participants, during the conversation about how they cope with these experiences. Coping from many participants means distancing from the experience, imposing preventive measures from the negative influence of grief. However, as some participants suggested, this 'armour' will only offer a moderate protection, meaning that it's almost impossible not to be affected somehow by grief.

> So, when you wear that uniform, that is an armour, it's really weird. You have this armour that protects you slightly and the way you manage your grief.
>
> (Mary, Sister)

Mary also described her way of coping as holding all the memories in an imaginary cupboard, with many drawers inside her mind. Sorting these memories suggests that she does not want to lose them, they've become part of who she is.

> I've got lots of cupboards in my brain, for my thoughts and feelings, different doors. One for example have a door for death, where it might sound very strange, but this is how I cope. So, all the deaths I have experienced at work will go into this cupboard. When I have a new death, there's a box for every child or adult. This is how I manage traumatic events at work, this is my way of handling it.
>
> (Mary, Sister)

One of the most common methods of coping described by almost all the participants was talking about the experience, by verbalising, expressing their thoughts and emotions. Many of them preferred to speak about these intimate feelings with someone very close to them, their spouse, partner, parent, or a very close friend. In the same time others preferred to talk about these experiences at work, with a colleague, protecting their personal circle from the effects of these traumatic events. Other times talking was combined with sport or physical activity, such as jogging or running, helping participants to relieve the accumulated stress.

> Straight away I come home and speak especially to my loved ones and running, I really enjoy running.
>
> (Andrew, Consultant)

> So, how I manage things. I tend to ring my mum if there's been a death and I cry a lot. That's how I overcome sadness I just cry. I talk a lot; I need to talk about it.
>
> (Mary, Sister)

> I think my personal coping mechanism is to go home and see my family and then I get upset or unload, but I can't really see doing that at work.
>
> (Margaret, Sister)

In addition, to talking to family or friends, participants discussed various professional methods that they use to access support. Some used TRIM (Trauma Risk Management), a service provided by the hospital to assess the psychological impact on staff of the exposure to distressing situations. This service is open to everyone affected by an incident and works by help exploring how the individual is coping after a traumatic event, potentially offering additional support. Other participants mentioned talking to a psychologist, a service offered during the COVID-19 pandemic by the hospital. While some welcomed this service, many participants did not feel comfortable discussing their emotions with a 'stranger over the phone'.

The most common professional support accessed by staff were hot and cold debriefs. A hot debrief is a gathering with the team involved in the death of a patient, including all specialities, whom in some form cared for that patient. A cold debrief is a similar meeting, but it happens a few weeks after the event. Participants were divided in which might be a better method for offering support. Most participants agreed that the advantage of these meetings is that they bring everyone involved together, but a disadvantage could be that not everyone might have a voice, or that the meeting could be dominated by the opinions of a few people, particularly if it is not led by an experienced person.

> We do debrief so once the patient passed away, we would if we can, do a hot debrief, one that is pretty much soon after the event. Unfortunately, with ED we have patients coming through the door all the time, so we normally do a

> cold debrief. But if I am honest, we are not very good in doing debriefs in our department.
>
> (Christine, Senior Sister)

> We have a debrief after we have a particularly traumatic case. But sometimes I'm not sure if that's enough.
>
> (David, Senior Charge Nurse)

> I think personally stirring up emotions in cold debrief is not useful but discussing things in a hot debrief is very helpful.
>
> (John, Junior Doctor)

Some participants also reported other forms of dealing with such traumatic events, such as the use of humour or playing video games, helping them manage the associated anxiety and stress.

> I think working in the Emergency Department … means that you have a slightly weird sense of humour and sometimes you can say things that are inappropriate for some people but not for you.
>
> (Rachel, Advanced Clinical Practitioner)

> Sometimes when it comes to dealing with stress, I am into games, sometimes just shooting some people. I don't think I need large amount of coping as I've seen enough death and I know how to pause, stop when it becomes horrible, and I need to move on.
>
> (Nicholas, Consultant)

Another form of coping with the death experience was noted in the language used by the HCPs interviewed, who were often using euphemisms when referring to death. Euphemisms are metaphors or analogies, often used to convey something considered too direct, without saying a specific word. The word 'death', and their different variations, are terms that in certain situations could be interpreted to be too 'painful', and as such are often cushioned in more indirect or protective language (Kessler, 2019). There could be several reasons why people choose to use euphemisms. Often euphemisms for death and dying are used to protect the person speaking the words or those hearing them. Avoiding using these direct terms could provide comfort, despite the grief of the situation (Naik, 2013). Avoiding being rude and offensive could be another reason, with the objective of not increasing the hurt and pain of someone by being too direct or blunt. While death and dying are a natural part of life, they could make some people feel uncomfortable or anxious. Using a milder language may feel easier and less traumatic under some circumstances (Krawczyk and Gallagher, 2016). Sometimes using euphemisms reflects our own grief feelings, as death is final, and saying it out loud can be difficult, especially if we experience a struggle to cope with this experience (Collins et al., 2018).

As discussed in an earlier chapter, according to some grieving models, denial represents a step in this complex process (Kubler-Ross, 1969). Using euphemisms could be a manifestation of a partial denial, as when using the word 'dead' makes it difficult to deny the reality. Indirect language, as a short-term coping mechanism, can sometimes be a helpful way to deal with the death experience mentally and emotionally (Collins et al., 2018). When spirituality represents an important aspect of someone's life and faith or a belief is central, the emphasis in death is the afterlife (Kessler, 2019). As observed in the answers given by certain participants in this study, this was not an avoidance tactic at all, but rather a shared reminder of the comfort found in their faith.

HCPs may still find it challenging to speak about death and dying directly, despite working in an area where exposure to death is not unusual. Sometimes this happens when bad news is delivered in a gentle and tactful way, being driven by compassion and a desire to soften the blow. Other times, HCPs have little training on how to cope with the emotional impact of caring for patients who die, as such euphemisms are used as coping strategies (Krawczyk and Gallagher, 2016). Analysing participant's answers in my study, it was obvious that interviewees in their answers predominantly used the terms 'death', 'dead', 'die', 'died', and 'dying'. In case of three of the participants, these were the only terms used, avoiding any form of indirect language. However, in certain situations most of the participants used euphemism. The alternative terms to describe death and dying, in most of the cases were 'passing away' or 'passed away' and 'losing someone', 'lost someone', or simply 'loss'. On some very rare occasions, describing death as a spiritual event, or a transition to another form of (eternal) life, some participants used expressions to describe death and dying, such as 'being with God'.

When listening to the recorded interviews and during the transcribing process, it became obvious what went unnoticed during the interviews that often involuntarily I've used the same euphemisms in the conversation or when asking a question from a participant. When I reflected on this phenomenon, I noted the followings in my own researcher journal:

> Using the same words for 'death' in the interview as my participant, such as 'passing away' surprised me completely, as I wasn't aware of it, until I've listened to the recording. I was so immersed in the conversation, feeling what the participant felt, displaying compassion towards an experience that visibly still affected them, that I simply mirrored their choice of words. Clearly, this detailed description of their experience made an emotional and psychological impact on me as well.

One of the typical occasions when participants used euphemisms was when they've described a death experience in the family or of someone in a very close relationship with them. Often these experiences served as reminders when exposed to a death in the ED that featured similar characteristics. Christine, when describing her motivation of becoming a nurse, mentions her grandmother's death, using euphemism:

> My grandma was a nurse, and she passed away in January of the last year of my studies, so she didn't see me qualifying, which was really upsetting at the time obviously. I hope I made her proud.
>
> (Christine, Senior Sister)

Another moment of switching to indirect language is when the deceased patient, 'suddenly becomes a person' for clinical staff. Zoe, when describing her experience of meeting a deceased patient's family, also cushioned the word 'death':

> … with nursing, it's something that is going to happen, you are going to lose a patient and it's hard. And here with us, I think the hardest part is when you get to be involved with the family, because you have to know them, and you get to know the person left behind.
>
> (Zoe, Senior Sister)

The stories told by the participants, related to their death experiences, carried certain features that made them memorable and unforgettable. One of these features was the patient's age. This was another prominent example of euphemisms being used:

> So earlier this year there was an 18-year-old girl, who was in a boat crush, and she came in very poorly and despite everything we did, we couldn't save her … so sadly she passed away.
>
> (Margaret, Sister)

The death of a child, especially if the circumstances were traumatic, very often triggered the same effect of softening the account, with the choice of words used to describe it. Julie is using three different euphemisms in the same story, when describing her experience:

> She came in as a traumatic cardiac arrest and I was looking to this little girl while they were doing CPR, cannulate, taking bloods, who has done nothing wrong in her life and is just hanging to life. She passed away and it was horrific because the parents weren't there only her auntie. … I didn't understand how a beautiful girl who didn't do anything wrong in her life could lost her life so tragically. She had a brilliant life ahead of her, but because of a silly mistake that somebody made, took her life and I said it's not fair.
>
> (Julie, Healthcare Assistant)

Table 7.1 Frequency of euphemisms used for death, dead, die(d), and dying

Study participant (pseudonym)	*Occurrence of the terms:* death, dead, die(d), and dying	*Occurrence of the terms:* passing(passed) away	*Occurrence of the terms:* losing, loss, and lost (someone)
Christine	47	15	0
Erica	19	1	1
Isaac	34	1	3
Rachel	14	3	3
John	15	8	2
Andrew	20	0	0
Mary	49	1	2
Robert	30	0	0
Nicholas	37	2	0
William	18	4	0
Margaret	17	0	4
Annabelle	2	3	1
Charlie	39	8	0
Adam	56	0	0
Julie	42	15	2
David	38	1	0
Zoe	17	4	9
Total:	**494**	**66**	**27**

Lastly, another typical example of avoiding the word 'death' was when participants were willing to express their empathy in a situation. Charlie describes a very emotional episode from his practice using the same euphemism as his colleagues:

> I remember, not this Christmas, but the Christmas before, someone was brought in, who was palliative, end-of-life, and the family didn't want to come in on Christmas Day. And this poor patient ended up passing away with staff around him, but you know, alone, in a Resus Room.
>
> (Charlie, Healthcare Assistant)

The type and frequency of occurrence for the various euphemisms used by the participants of the study, during the interviews, are listed in Table 7.1.

Learning from death

One of the significant observations, that most of the study participants made, was that death is still some sort of 'taboo', something that most people, including HCPs, feel uncomfortable talking about. Being exposed to death regularly caused clinical staff to be willing to talk about death more openly, and by doing so, to 'normalise death'.

> The first part is we need to acknowledge it, we must talk about, be open about it, because horrible things will happen. Death is a normal process at the end of the day, it happens to us all … I think that we just need to normalize death more and I think in the ED we are in a privileged position where we can support each other and make a difference.
>
> (Andrew, Consultant)

An observation made by many participants was the motivation to pursue a 'good death', a dignified death by implementing changes in their clinical practice. Participants clearly expressed that the way they view patient care is different because of these experiences, for example, often not willing to preserve life at all costs but to act in the best interests of their patients.

> Thinking now as a [senior member of staff], seeing a lot of death has impacted me in pursuing a good, dignified death where it's appropriate, things like DNACPR [Do Not Attempt Cardio-Pulmonary Resuscitation], treatment escalation plans, that sort of things.
>
> (Nicholas, Consultant)

> In terms of how I changed my practice, hasn't really because, care is care, nursing is nursing, but with these experiences I think it gave me more inside knowledge on how my brain works and possibly how are we optimizing the care for our patients.
>
> (David, Senior Charge Nurse)

> I don't really like when people had lots of interventions up to the point of them dying. Because for me it feels like it's not as dignified. It's hard, it's not an easy balance.
>
> (Andrew, Consultant)

Another element observed by participants in how their attitude to patient care has changed is related to improving communication and building a relationship both with patients and families. Family relations, for many HCPs, become a priority alongside clinical interventions, as end-of-life care provided in the ED will be remembered by families.

> I would say you get different patients in A&E and some of them will pass away, you just make sure you always treat your patients with good care, making sure they are not in any pain, always speak with them and make a rapport with them. I think supporting the families is a big thing and from a personal experience you remember that situation.
>
> (Margaret, Sister)

When asked about what training they have received to help them cope with the death experience, healthcare assistants and nurses confirmed that they either have not received any education or just something very basic. Doctors confirmed that it is part of their training to learn how to break bad news or conduct difficult conversations. When asked if they would prefer to have training sessions that would better prepare them for the psychological and emotional impact of the experience or other aspects of looking after the dying patient, participants had mixed views. Some suggested that exposure to death experiences is the only way to gain understanding and that should happen in a safe environment with support that helps processing these traumatic events. Others however expressed that they would prefer a better preparation, discussion on certain aspects of death and dying, so that they can follow evidence-based practice, instead of departmental tradition.

> I guess that comes from experience and I don't know if anybody telling me about it would have changed what it was like, because for me I am quite a visual person, even if someone would have told me about it.
>
> (Rachel, Advanced Clinical Practitioner)

> I don't think you can prepare yourself prior to death. Because every family is different, every death is different.
>
> (Mary, Sister)

> Through your career you will see horrific things especially if you are in A&E, so why can't we do a half a day on bereavement care? The other day I was talking with someone about having last offices and they thought that's all about wrapping up people and getting them ready. Why people are not taught how to properly look after the dead, because at the end of the day this is just part of our training.
>
> (Julie, Healthcare Assistant)

Many of the participants were in leadership roles, as sisters or charge nurses, consultants, or in roles with the added responsibility of managing a team. In the event of a patient death, most senior staff described that they would make their teams' needs a priority, when dealing with this experience, sometimes delaying, or postponing coping with their own feelings. Almost all members of staff in a leadership position expressed a sense of responsibility for their team, often finding that focusing on other peoples' needs helped them better cope with their own emotions.

> I think you clocked up experience, and you understand what their concerns are about. I think you can offer useful advice at that time. And I think that is part of what a leader is. Looking after people that he works with.
>
> (Robert, Advanced Clinical Practitioner)

> As it affected me, it put things into perspective to see how much it affected someone else. For me it's actually quite a positive thing, to go and sit down and explain what we did and why we did it. So, it's very positive to help someone else.
>
> (Andrew, Consultant)

Almost all participants expressed that they would like to continue their professional career in ED, or they would like to embrace these experiences, and expand their professional role or learning. Some talked about how dealing with death helped them to pursue a career in clinical education, while others wanted to become more involved in supporting and training fellow nurses, or pursuing a role in palliative, end-of-life, or bereavement care and services.

> Helping and teaching our staff drove me towards education, which I am doing part-time. So, this was something I think might have influenced me.
>
> (Isaac, Charge Nurse)

> I think because my experience was so dramatic for me, in the future I'd like to do something to help other people that have similar experiences, other nurses or members of staff.
>
> (Erica, Nurse)

> Later in life I can see myself continuing in bereavement services or maybe end-of-life care.
>
> (Julie, Healthcare Assistant)

Participants expressed feelings of gratitude to have the opportunity to work in the ED, considering it a 'humbling experience' or something that 'feels right' for them, despite witnessing death regularly, which most of the time didn't contribute to be an influence in changing the course of their career prospects.

> With my career, I just want to carry on. I think it's a humbling experience and it's always changing you as a person. I always look at the positive things with every experience.
>
> (Zoe, Senior Sister)

> Some of my friends want to be surgeons because they can go to theatre... When I'm in the Resus Room supporting people in that acute instance, it just feels right to me.
>
> (John, Junior Doctor)

Discussion: the influence of death in the Emergency Department

Participants of my empirical study experienced various changes personally and professionally as a response to their experiences of death in the ED. This included changes to how they view life itself and interpret the world surrounding them, or changes in clinical practices, attitudes, and their relationship with the dying patient and their family. Kuek et al. (2020) argue that individual experiences that are poorly processed, including those with death and dying, which are immersed in professional, emotional, ethical, and psychological challenges for those working in healthcare, can have a major influence on how HCPs deal with their choices and decisions. Studies also suggest that professional identity, individual personhood, and even patient care are impacted by how well HCPs can manage the death and dying experiences (White and Meeker, 2019; Terakado and Matsushima, 2015; Diehl et al., 2021; Zheng et al., 2022). My study confirms that HCPs' priorities, behaviours, and relationships have been impacted in numerous ways by their death experience in the ED.

Ho et al. (2022) interviewed senior palliative care and oncology nurses in Singapore and aimed to understand the impact of death and dying on the nurses' personhood, principles, values, beliefs, and professional identities, in correlation with the Ring Theory of Personhood. Inspired by Confucian ethics, the Ring Theory of Personhood describes personhood as having an 'Innate', 'Individual', 'Relational', and 'Societal' domain, each containing specific values, beliefs, morals, and norms (Radha Krishna and Alsuwaigh, 2015). The 'Innate' domain deals with gender, religious, moral, ethical, and cultural values, the 'Individual' domain holds the personality and the personal values, whilst the 'Relational' and 'Societal' domains incorporate any family or wider society-related expectations and values (Radha Krishna and Alsuwaigh, 2015). A visual representation of the Ring Theory of Personhood can be found in Figure 7.1.

Ho et al. (2022) described the impact of death and dying on nurses, using three themes: 'Identity formation', 'Identity conflict and its influences', and 'Identity refinement' in relation to the Ring Theory of Personhood. 'Identity formation' identified significant changes experienced by nurses at the beginning of their career or when they've entered the field of palliative care or oncology. These changes were ranging from the development of empathy and a dignity-focused care for the dying, to the alleviation of the fear of death, strengthening religious beliefs or weighing life

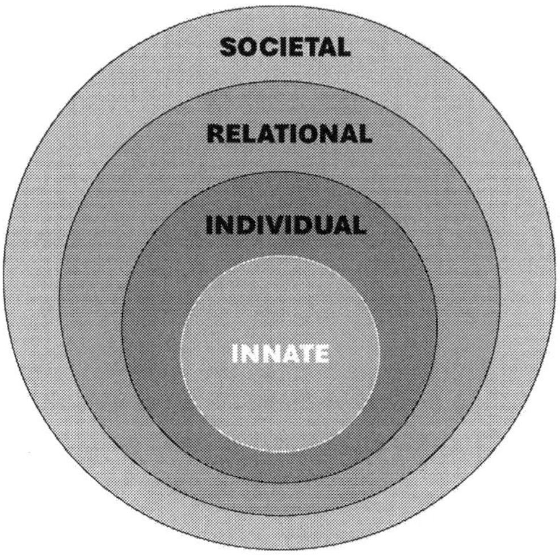

Figure 7.1 Visual representation of the 'Ring Theory of Personhood'.

choices differently. 'Identity conflict and its influences' described how the death and dying experience created some conflicts among values, beliefs, and principles, and influenced nurses' professional and personal identity. Finally, 'Identity refinement' discussed how these conflicts are addressed, to maintain a stable, balanced identity. These included principles of coping and changes in family relations, work-life balance, or parenting methods, but also a change in how nurses were defining a 'good life' and a 'good death' (Ho et al., 2022). Participants of my study also reflect on how the death experience had a gradual influence, on their views about life and death, changed their family priorities, the way they express gratitude in their everyday life, or how they allow themselves to express their own emotions in front of others. A visual representation of these three major stages can be found in Figure 7.2.

Participants of my empirical study talked about how an emotional investment is required when dealing with dying patients and how this experience triggers a series of feelings from sadness to failure, requiring from them an emotional labour. Emotional labour that accompanies a crisis in the ED can be described as demanding, an attitude that requires sensitivity when acting and reacting in a traumatic situation (Bennett et al., 2005). Hochschild (1983) describes emotional labour as managing or altering emotions to maintain an external display that helps others feel supported, comfortable, and emotionally secure. A link between caring for terminally ill patients, patients transitioning from active treatment into palliative care, or patients in pain and experiencing loss, and emotional labour in nursing, was clearly identified (James, 1992; Smith, 1992; Kelly, 2000), alongside the need for an emotional connectedness and related regulations strategies, between HCPs and their patients (Bender et al., 2021; Kimbell et al., 2020). Bailey et al. (2011) argue that a distancing behaviour in ED nurses is often the result of an inability to manage this emotional labour; however, this coping mechanism can be more stressful on the long term.

Hunsaker et al. (2015) in his qualitative survey study, conducted with the involvement of approximately 700 emergency nurses in the United States, argue that compassion fatigue can be defined as the negative consequences of having a strong, personal, empathic orientation, while working with a significant number of traumatised individuals. On the contrary, compassion satisfaction occurs when

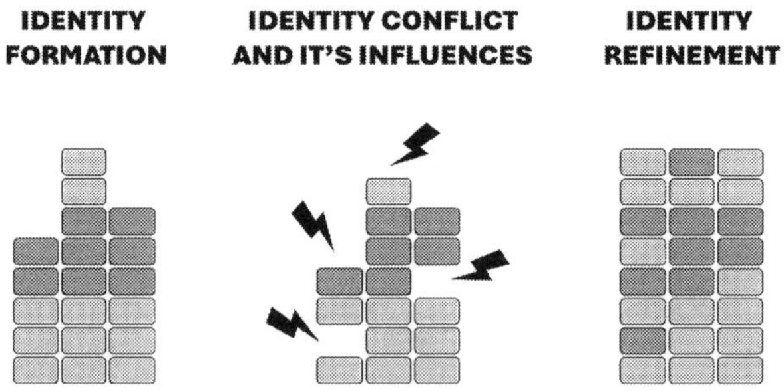

Figure 7.2 The three stages of the death and dying impact on nurses (adapted from Ho et al., 2022).

the emergency nurse feels a sense of connection with their patients and a sense of achievement in the care provided for these patients (Hunsaker et al., 2015). Another US qualitative survey study aimed on emergency nurses, investigating the prevalence of secondary traumatic stress (STS), suggests that exposure to human suffering has a potentially negative consequence with a profound effect on emergency nurses' health (Dominguez-Gomez and Rutledge, 2009). STS refers to exposure to a person who is traumatised or suffering rather than exposure to a traumatic event itself, resulting in an emotional disequilibrium (Dominguez-Gomez and Rutledge, 2009). The study reported at least one STS symptom in 85% of the nurses exposed to traumatic events, while 33% met the criterion for a diagnosis of STS. Symptoms such as irritability, intrusive thoughts, emotional numbing, sleeping disorders, diminished activity level, and avoidance of patients were the most reported by the participating emergency nurses (Dominguez-Gomez and Rutledge, 2009). Similarly to the findings of these studies, participants interviewed in my research were reporting on a wide range of emotions, ranging from sadness, feeling upset, fear, for some of them causing disturbances in their sleeping or eating habits.

HCPs interviewed in my empirical study talked about experiencing individual emotions and the importance of acknowledging them, yet as a team, often sharing these feelings. The study of Kostka et al. (2021) surveyed 160 Polish nurses in a municipal hospital and reached to the conclusion that there are several emotions shared among them, when dealing with death. The most common shared emotions were helplessness (62.5% of the respondents), compassion (54.17%), sadness (54.17%), and depression (41.67%). Feeling helpless was a common shared emotion reported by my study, which often occurred in case of a sudden and unexpected, or traumatic death event.

Coping with death was described by the participants of my empirical study in various forms, from numbing or internalising feelings, and using an 'armour' for protection, up to talking about their experiences with family members or accessing professional support services. As discussed in the earlier chapters, a traumatic event can be defined as a powerful, extreme, or severe situation, circumstances, or chain of events, able to overwhelm through its intensity a person's ability to cope, which may result in unusually strong emotional, cognitive, or behavioural reactions (Meichenbaum, 1994). ED is almost constantly confronted with severe injuries, death, suicide, and suffering (Bennett et al., 2005; McFarlane and Bryant, 2007). During confrontation with a traumatic event, ED nurses often adopt avoidance as a coping strategy (Crabbe et al., 2004). Avoidance, which can manifest, for example, in distraction, in short terms can have the benefit for an emergency worker to be able to go on functioning. Nevertheless, in longer terms this may hinder the recovery process and can therefore lead to the development of severe psychosomatic symptoms (Clohessy and Ehlers, 1999). Wearing a uniform was often seen by the participants of my study as wearing an 'armour' that protects them from the effects of the death experience. While some suggested to use 'shielding' as an avoidant coping mechanism, others reflected on allowing themselves to become vulnerable in front of others as seeing kindness, empathy, and compassion of a high importance, because of their death experiences. Yet, other participants in my study reported developing an emotional numbness over the years and almost not 'feeling anything' when encountering death. Similarly, Bailey et al. (2011) reached to the conclusion that avoidance is used by HCPs as a 'shield' to protect themselves from the negative influences and upsetting feelings associated with witnessing death, especially if dying has a slow trajectory.

The study of Adriaenssens et al. (2012) surveyed more than 300 nurses in 15 Belgian hospitals, and indicates that during the emergency care interventions, ED nurses can adopt three major types of coping mechanism: emotion-oriented, task-oriented, and avoidant. Emotion-oriented coping strategies are self-oriented emotional reactions to reduce stress, usually not successful in nurses. These reactions range from blaming oneself for being too emotional, angry, tense, self-preoccupied to simply fantasising (Adriaenssens et al., 2012). Task-oriented coping mechanisms are often seen as successful because they require an attitude of control, influence, commitment, and resilience (Adriaenssens et al., 2012). Avoidant coping strategies, such as denial, wishful thinking, emotional suppression of intrusion, and mental disengagement, are described as unhelpful by ED staff, as proved to have long-term negative effect on wellbeing (Adriaenssens et al., 2012). Some of the participants of my study reported some unhealthy coping mechanisms, such as excessive alcohol consumption or physical exercise, which didn't help managing these experiences. One participant described their avoidant coping strategy, as using an imaginary cupboard, where memories are stored, while another participant was using FPS (first-person shooter) videogames to cope.

Peters et al. (2013) argue that ED offers little or no time to cope and that nurses with a longer experience will adopt more efficient coping strategies, compared to their less experienced colleagues. Participants of my empirical study often expressed their frustration about their inability to take a break after a death experience, being required to take the next patient, which jeopardised their own wellbeing and the quality of care provided. Kostka et al. (2021) found that the level of coping with death among HCPs was directly dependent on the level of seniority. Nurses with the least time spent in the department experienced the highest rate of helplessness, while those with a longer period of service talked about higher capability to overcome consequences.

Giles et al. (2019) surveyed 211 Australian ED nurses and concluded that debriefs are an efficient support for coping with death; however, due to time pressures they are often missed, organised several weeks after the event, or they are not led by an expert, as such they often prove not to be helpful. Gerace et al. (2020) reached to the same conclusion that the inability to debrief is one of the factors that lead to an end-of-life care in the ED, that is not satisfying for HCPs, the patient, and their family. Debriefs were reported in my empirical study, as being very efficient tools in supporting HCPs; however, timing and the skills of those leading these debriefs were seen by participants as crucial.

The need to talk about death more openly, the willingness to pursue a 'good death', to improve communication with the deceased patient's family, the provision of training and preparation for facing death, and the career perspectives influenced by death, for participants in my study represented the cornerstones for HCPs, to learn from their death experiences. Kübler-Ross (1969) argues that the subject of death historically was an uncomfortable topic, yet individuals are often eager to talk honestly about death, especially when that involves unresolved family issues, or it simply means expressing their own sadness. One of the reasons to keep the topic of death as a taboo, according to Chen et al. (2019), is related to death anxiety, described as the fear or panic, that someone's experiencing, when they are faced with their own mortality. A qualitative study conducted by Üzar-Özçetin et al. (2021) among 28 final-year Turkish nursing student about their experiences of talking about death with terminally ill patients concluded that participants typically adopt three attitudes in such situations. They will either question their own competency and refrain from initiating the conversation, a similar avoidance because of the assumption and prejudice of causing harm to patients, or they are willing to discuss the topic but would benefit from experiential learning opportunities to develop the required skills. My study also reports that some HCPs find it difficult to openly talk about death expectation with their patients, as it goes against the core ethos of saving lives and improving patient's wellbeing.

The study of Bergenholtz et al. (2020) interviewing patients and their relatives in a Danish hospital found that patients would be willing for HCPs to discuss death and end-of-life with them if that is done in a dignified environment, with a family member present and in an empathetic, compassionate manner. Participants of my study acknowledged as well that death is a topic they often feel uncomfortable talking about; however, they see it as an opportunity to learn through these conversations, how to better deal with such experiences. Providing a 'good death' has a similar importance as maintaining a quality of life in terminally ill patients (Smith, 2000). According to Steinhauser et al. (2000), a 'good death' in a hospital setting is determined by the following factors: control of symptoms, preparation for death, a sense of 'closure' or 'completion' in life, and a good relationship with the HCPs, with an emphasis for patients on retaining control over their own destiny. Participants interviewed in my empirical study reported that one form of offering a 'good death' is by knowing when to stop any active treatment that proves to be futile. There is great debate about determining what constitutes, a futile treatment, a beneficent outcome and who should make this decision, yet there is a consensus that the question reaches beyond physiological measures, and psychological, social, economic, religious, familial, and legal aspects are also important (Schneiderman, 1994; Brody, 1994; Veatch, 1994). A futile treatment should be balanced in the view of the individual's goals to be achieved and the possible success rate of the treatment which in their view is acceptable (Faber-Langendoen, 1991).

Participants of my study expressed the importance of improving communication with family members, because of their experience with death. Peters et al. (2013) suggest that a therapeutic communication style will help the patient and its family to express with more ease their wishes, but also to accept the inevitable and find comfort, and a sense of closure at the end of their life (Peters et al., 2013). Giles et al. (2019) argue that difficult and sensitive conversations should not be delayed with patients and their families, as that can become an obstacle for an early understanding of the dying patient and their family needs. Participants of my study often reported how the death experiences helped them to improve their communication style and be more attentive to the family needs. Senior HCPs in a leadership role, interviewed in my study, both consultants and senior sisters or charge nurses, expressed the importance of offering support to their team, when they go through witnessing a traumatic event. Adriaenssens et al. (2012) argue that social support from the supervisor, in the view of emergency nurses, had close links to reduced psychological distress and somatic complaints, while adequate support from colleagues was associated with less fatigue. Hunsaker et al. (2015) suggest that support from managers, shared decision-making processes, and recognising nurses' contributions to practice are directly related to increased nurse retention, increased job satisfaction, and reduced staff turnover. A supportive manager will engage in a positive relationship with clinical staff in the ED, such leaders having a fundamental role in the successful development of safe, positive, and open professional environments.

The importance of preparation, trainings, and exposure to death experiences, for the purpose of practical learning, was regularly argued by the participants of my study. Whitehead et al. (2010) argue that training programmes focusing on preparing staff for the death experience and the development of skills in providing spiritual care have a positive effect in nurses' attitudes towards death. Bailey et al. (2011) suggest that one of the important supports ED staff should receive is professional training in end-of-life care and dealing with the psychological and emotional aspect of care for the dying patient. In Bailey et al.'s (2011) view, this professional preparation for the death experiences should start at university, rather than the ED, both at undergraduate and postgraduate level. The study conducted by Mar Díaz-Cortés et al. (2018), among ED nurses and doctors, found that professional trainings surrounding the death experience will not only improve HCPs' capability in coping with traumatising events, but will also support their decision-making processes and the management of their own emotions. Participants of my study had mixed feelings about an education programme focusing on the death experience. While some argued that it would be beneficial not only to understand processes surrounding death but also to learn how to cope and access support services, others suggested that a training can't prepare someone for the death experience, as such they recommended regular, safe exposure to death as a way of practical learning.

Majority of the participants asked about their career plans during the interviews of my study, reflected on staying in the ED, despite their experiences with death, some even pursuing career goals in palliative care or bereavement services. Tavakoli et al. (2018) surveyed 709 emergency nurses in ten hospitals in Iran and concluded that 76.1% of them are experiencing moderate levels of burnout. Several studies discovered a link between the burnout of HCPs, a work-related stress syndrome resulting from chronic exposure to job stress and career choice regret (Dyrbye et al., 2018; Chen, 2014; Shanafelt et al., 2009). The study of Wu and Volker (2009) interviewed 14 Taiwanese hospice nurses, from six different hospices, about their experiences with death and dying, and found that many nurses,

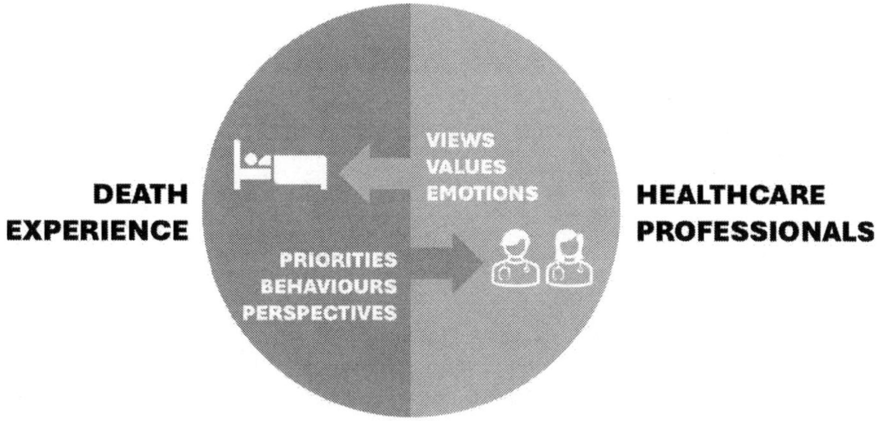

Figure 7.3 The dual interaction between healthcare professionals and the death experience.

because of constantly being exposed to death and grief, started questioning their career choice and making plans about staying or leaving their field of work. My study contradicts these findings, as none of the interviewed participants experienced career choice regret; on the contrary, many of them were willing to pursue a career or be more involved in bereavement or end-of-life care.

Experiencing death in the ED can be the catalyst for a series of changes in HCPs, both personally and professionally, including their priorities, behaviours, or relationships. Managing death in the ED requires an emotional labour from clinical staff, some experiencing professional grief, often a sense of failure, but valuing kindness and empathy, while sharing many emotions with the rest of the team. Coping with the death experience can range from shielding to the use of humour, talking about the experience, and using professional support services, such as debriefs, are among the most common forms. Aiming for a 'good death', improving communication with families, theoretical and practical preparation for the death experience, and pursuing certain careers are all part of the learning process from the death experience in the ED. This book argues that both the individual and the death experience interact with each other. HCPs will shape the death experience through their values, views about death and their emotional investment, while the death experience will influence HCPs' perspectives, priorities, or behaviours. This dual interaction is illustrated in Figure 7.3.

Reference list

Adriaenssens, J., de Gucht, V., Maes, S. (2012). The impact of traumatic events on emergency room nurses: Findings from a questionnaire survey. *International Journal of Nursing Studies*, 49(11), pp. 1411–1422.

Bailey, C., Murphy, R., Porock, D. (2011). Trajectories of end-of-life care in the Emergency Department. *Annals of Emergency Medicine*, 57(4), pp. 362–369.

Bender, A.E., Berg, K.A., Miller, E.K., Evans, K.E., Holmes, M.R. (2021). "Making sure we are all okay": Healthcare workers' strategies for emotional connectedness during the COVID-19 pandemic. *Clinical Social Work Journal*, 49(4), pp. 445–455.

Bennett, P., Williams, Y., Page, N., Hood, K., Woollard, M., Vetter, N. (2005). Associations between organizational and incident factors and emotional distress in emergency ambulance personnel. *British Journal of Clinical Psychology*, 44(6–2), pp. 215–226.

Bergenholtz, H., Missel, M., Timm, H. (2020). Talking about death and dying in a hospital setting - A qualitative study of the wishes for end-of-life conversations from the perspective of patients and spouses. *BMC Palliative Care*, 19(1), p. 168.

Brody, H. (1994). The physician's role in determining futility. *Journal of American Geriatric Society*, 42(8), pp. 875–878.

Chen, J.S., Wen, F.H., Chou, W.C., Hsieh, C.H., Chang, W.C., Tang, S.T. (2019). Terminally ill cancer patients' distinct symptomfunctional patterns/states are differentially associated with their accurate prognostic awareness in the last six months of life. *Journal of Palliative Medicine*, 22(7), pp. 782–789.

Chen, X. (2014). Study of burnout status and influencing factors of clinical graduate students. *Health Vocational Education*, 32(20), pp. 114–116.

Clohessy, S., Ehlers, A. (1999). PTSD symptoms, response to intrusive memories and coping in ambulance service workers. *British Journal of Clinical Psychology*, 38(3), pp. 251–265.

Collins, A., McLachlan, S., Philip, J. (2018). How should we talk about palliative care, death and dying? A qualitative study exploring perspectives from caregivers of people with advanced cancer. *Palliative Medicine*, 32(4), pp. 861–869.

Crabbe, J., Bowley, D., Boffard, K., Alexander, D., Klein, S. (2004). Are health professionals getting caught in the crossfire? The personal implications of caring for trauma victims. *Emergency Medicine Journal*, 21, pp. 568–572.

Diehl, E., Rieger, S., Letzel, S., Schablon, A., Nienhaus, A., Escobar Pinzon, L.C., Dietz, P. (2021). Burdens, resources, health and wellbeing of nurses working in general and specialised palliative care in Germany - Results of a nationwide cross-sectional survey study. *BMC Nursing*, 20(1), p. 162.

Dominguez-Gomez, E., Rutledge, D.N. (2009). Prevalence of secondary traumatic stress among emergency nurses. *Journal of Emergency Nursing*, 35(3), pp. 199–204.

Dyrbye, L.N., Burke, S.E., Hardeman, R.R., Herrin, J., Wittlin, N.M., Yeazel, M. (2018). Association of clinical specialty with symptoms of burnout and career choice regret among us resident physicians. *Journal of American Medical Association*, 320(11), pp. 1114–1130.

Faber-Langendoen, K. (1991). Resuscitation of patients with metastatic cancer. Is transient benefit still futile? *Archives of Internal Medicine*, 151(2), pp. 235–239.

Gerace, A., Giles, T., Breaden, K., Hammad, K., Drummond, C., Bradley, S.L., Muir-Cochrane, E. (2020). Nurses' perceptions of dealing with death in the Emergency Department. *Collegian*, 28(1), pp. 71–80.

Giles, T.M., Hammad, K., Breaden, K., Drummond, C., Bradley, S.L., Gerace, A., Muir-Cochrane, E. (2019). Nurses' perceptions and experiences of caring for patients who die in the Emergency Department setting. *International Emergency Nursing*, 47, p. 100789. Available at: https://pubmed.ncbi.nlm.nih.gov/31495727

Ho, C.Y., Lim, N., Ong, Y.T., Lee, A.S.I., Chiam, M., Gek, G.P.L., Sarraf-Yazdi, S., Mason, S., Krishna, L. (2022). The impact of death and dying on the personhood of senior nurses at the National Cancer Centre Singapore (NCCS): A qualitative study. *BMC Palliative Care*, 21, p. 83. Available at: https://doi.org/10.1186/s12904-022-00974-9

Hochschild, A.R. (1983). *The managed heart. Commercialization of human feeling*. Berkeley: University of California Press.
Hunsaker, S., Chen, H.C., Maughan, D., Heaston, S. (2015). Factors that influence the development of compassion fatigue, burnout, and compassion satisfaction in Emergency Department nurses. *Journal of Nursing Scholarship*, 47(2), pp. 186–194.
James, N. (1992). Care organisation, physical labour and emotional labour. *Sociology of Health and Illness*, 14(4), pp. 488–505.
Kelly, B. (2000). Terminally ill cancer patient's wish to hasten death. *Palliative Medicine*, 16(4), pp. 339–345.
Kessler, D. (2019). *Finding meaning. The sixth stage of grief.* New York: Scribner.
Kimbell, L.M., Boudreaux, E.D., Chimowitz, H., Liu, G., Cyr, E., Kimall, E. (2020). What do Emergency Department physicians and nurses feel? A qualitative study of emotions, triggers, regulation strategies, and effects on patient care. *British Medical Journal Quality and Safety*, 29(10), pp. 1–2.
Krawczyk, M., Gallagher, R. (2016). Communicating prognostic uncertainty in potential end-of-life contexts: Experiences of family members. *BMC Palliative Care*, 15, p. 59. Available at: https://doi.org/10.1186/s12904-016-0133-4
Kostka, A.M., Borodzicz, A., Krzemińska, S.A. (2021). Feelings and emotions of nurses related to dying and death of patients – A pilot study. *Psychology Research and Behavior Management*, 14, pp. 705–717.
Kübler-Ross, E. (1969). *On death and dying.* New York: The Macmillan Company.
Kuek, J.T.Y., Ngiam, L.X.L., Kamal, N.H.A., Chia, J.L., Chan, N.P.X., Abdurrahman, A.B.H.M., Ho, C.Y., Tan, L.H.E., Goh, J.L., Khoo, M.S.Q., Ong, Y.T., Chiam, M., Chin, A.M.C., Mason, S., Krishna, L.K.R. (2020). The impact of caring for dying patients in intensive care units on a physician's personhood: A systematic scoping review. *The Journal of Philosophy, Ethics, and Humanities in Medicine*, 15(1), pp. 1–16.
Mar Díaz-Cortés, M.D., Granero-Molina, J., Hernández-Padilla, J.M., Rodríguez, R.P., Casado, M.C., Fernández-Sola, C. (2018). Promoting dignified end-of-life care in the Emergency Department: A qualitative study. *International Emergency Nursing*, 37, pp. 23–28.
McFarlane, A., Bryant, R. (2007). Post-traumatic stress disorder in occupational settings: Anticipating and managing the risk. *Occupational Medicine*, 57(6), pp. 404–410.
Meichenbaum, D. (1994). *A clinical handbook/practical therapist manual for assessing and treating adults with post-traumatic stress disorder*. Ontario: Institute Press.
Naik, S.B. (2013). Death in the hospital: Breaking the bad news to the bereaved family. *Indian Journal of Critical Care Medicine*, 17(3), pp. 178–181.
Peters, L., Cant, R., Payne, S., O'Connor, M., McDermott, F., Hood, K., Morphet, J., Shimoinaba, K. (2013). Emergency and palliative care nurses' levels of anxiety about death and coping with death: A questionnaire survey. *Australasian Emergency Nursing Journal*, 16(4), pp. 152–159.
Radha Krishna, L.K., Alsuwaigh, R. (2015). Understanding the fluid nature of personhood – The ring theory of personhood. *Medical Ethics Journal*, 29(3), pp. 171–181.
Schneiderman, L.J. (1994). The futility debate: Effective versus beneficial intervention. *Journal of American Geriatric Society*, 42(8), pp. 883–886.
Shanafelt, T.D., Balch, C.M., Bechamps, G.J. (2009). Burnout and career satisfaction among American surgeons. *Annals of Surgery*, 250(3), pp. 463–471.
Smith, P. (1992). *The emotional labour of nursing*. London: Edward Arnold.
Smith, R. (2000). A good death: An important aim for health services and us all. *British Medical Journal*, 320(7228), pp. 129–130.

Steinhauser, K.E., Christakis, N.A., Clipp, E.C., McNeilly, M., McIntyre, L., Tulsky, J.A. (2000). Factors considered important at the end of life by patients, family, physicians, and other care providers. *The Journal of the American Medical Association*, 284(19), pp. 2476–2482.

Tavakoli, N., Shaker, S.H., Soltani, S., Abbasi, M., Amini, M., Tahmasebi, A., Hosseini Kasnavieh, S.M. (2018). Job burnout, stress, and satisfaction among emergency nursing staff after health system transformation plan in Iran. *Emergency,* 6(1), p. e41.

Terakado, A., Matsushima, E. (2015). Work stress among nurses engaged in palliative care on general wards. *Psychooncology*, 24(1), pp. 63–69.

Zheng, R., Guo, Q., Dong, F., Gao, L. (2022). Death self-efficacy, attitudes toward death and burnout among oncology nurses: A multicenter cross-sectional study. *Cancer Nursing*, 45(2), pp. 388–396.

Üzar-Özçetin, Y.S., Hiçdurmaz, D., Öcalan, S. (2021). 'Who would even want to talk about death?' A qualitative study on nursing students' experiences of talking about death with terminally ill patients with cancer. *European Journal of Cancer Care*, 30(6), p. e13514.

Veatch, R.M. (1994). Why physicians cannot determine if care is futile. *Journal of American Geriatric Society*, 42(8), pp. 871–874.

White, D., Meeker, M.A. (2019). Guiding the process of dying: The personal impact on nurses. *Journal of Hospital Palliative Nursing*, 21(5), pp. 390–396.

Whitehead, P.B., Anderson, E.S., Redican, K.J., Stratton, R. (2010). Studying the effects of the end-of life nursing education consortium at the institutional level. *Journal of Hospice & Palliative Nursing*, 12(3), pp. 184–193.

Wu, H., Volker, D.L. (2009). Living with death and dying: The experience of Taiwanese hospice nurses. *Oncology Nursing Forum*, 36(5), pp. 578–584.

Chapter 8

Conclusion

Life after death

Deaths occurring in a hospital, particularly in the Emergency Department (ED), are events that have been commonly researched and analysed from the perspective of healthcare professionals (HCPs). One of the focuses in the current literature is on caring for the dying patient and exploring the physiological, psychological, and emotional impact and consequences of these experiences on health service providers. This book has discussed in detail, how both the individual, through their values and norms, and the death experience interact with each other, shaping this experience and its sense-making process.

One of the contributions this book makes to the wider knowledge base is by understanding how the death experiences of HCPs working in the ED are influenced by their personal norms and values, including the moral, ethical, cultural, social, and spiritual aspects. As values develop over time and are directly influenced by our gender, ethnicity, cultural and social circumstances, but also shaped by our experiences and interactions with others, they will establish moral standards and milestones as reference points, to guide us through our decisions. These values are not static or passive, they reflect in our actions, as gradually become part of our identity, creating a hierarchy that will help us understand ourselves and the reality surrounding us, influencing how death itself is perceived and interpreted. This book also concludes that deaths in the ED that occur unexpectedly, deaths of children and young adults, deaths that occurred during the early career or those that remind staff of the death of a family member, deaths that are traumatic, even 'horrifying' in their nature, are more likely to have an emotional, psychological, sometimes physiological influence on HCPs, that often could have lasting effects for years or even decades. Personal values will influence those characteristics of death in the ED, that makes them stand out, and often become memorable for HCPs, having sometimes a lasting impact on them as individuals and professionals. Values define what staff view as being a 'normal' or 'not normal', a 'fair' or 'unfair' death, or an 'acceptable' or 'unacceptable' loss, or how they will act and behave when caring for the dying. Making sense of death in the ED includes the language and euphemisms used by HCPs to describe death, often referring to it as a 'loss' or as the person 'passing away'. Personal values will also influence HCPs' chosen

DOI: 10.4324/9781032660912-8

coping mechanisms, the care provided for their patients or various interactions, perspectives, behaviours, or decisions made in their personal and professional life.

One of the implications for practice of the findings of this study relates to the development of new and improvement of existing education and training for ED staff, supporting their better preparation for the death experiences. While both medical and nursing higher education programmes in the UK provide a framework of teaching palliative and end-of-life related subjects and skills, including patient assessment, symptom control, or communication skills, these do not address some of the specific challenges of the death experience in the ED. Exposure to death experience of students during their training programme will depend on the practice placement allocations. One of the participants of the research study revealed that as a newly qualified nurse, had no personal or professional experience with witnessing death, prior of starting her career in the ED. Witnessing her first death in the ED had a considerable impact on her physiological and psychological wellbeing, feeling at that time unprepared for this experience.

Health Education England in partnership with the Leadership Alliance for the Care of Dying People, in its publication 'One Chance to Get It Right' (Leadership Alliance for the Care of Dying People, 2014), describes views and recommendations for improving people's experience of care in the last few days and hours of their life. One of the important statements the document makes is that "some staff caring for dying people do not have the skills and knowledge required to deliver care to high standards". Furthermore, it suggests that there is a responsibility in "ensuring staff have the experience and competence they need to do their jobs well. This includes making time and other resources available for staff to undergo professional development". The document recognises the importance of "communication skills, including empathy and recognising emotional response to stress and distress", and encourages integrating into learning modules that cover social care, bereavement, and spirituality, with an emphasis of consolidating and applying knowledge in different situations. While this document was published more than a decade ago, at the time of writing this book, nurse or healthcare assistant participants of my study reported that they have not received any formal training that would have prepared them for the complex task of caring for the dying patient, their families, and managing their own wellbeing as a result of this experience. Some initiatives are taking place to improve end-of-life care in the UK, through education programmes, such as the education improvement across the local health and care sector in Shropshire (NICE, 2018). However, these target mainly the hospice sector, rather than the acute or emergency care in NHS hospitals. Another innovative educational initiative is the 'Global Classroom', launched as a joint online training course, aimed on UK and US nursing students with the purpose of discussing various aspects of end-of-life care, including cultural differences of advance care planning and the role of HCPs (Bailey et al., 2017). Such initiatives can widen future HCPs' understanding of the complex phenomenon of dying, encouraging them to ask questions, raise concerns, respond effectively in difficult situations, from the start of their professional career.

Beyond the traditional subjects of palliative and end-of-life care, the training provided for HCPs, as part of their first 6–12 months of induction and preceptorship in the ED, should include learning about self-awareness and acknowledgement of their own values and norms, including social, cultural, spiritual, and moral values, and the influence these can have on their individual perception and experience of death. A similar topic could also be potentially added to the curriculum of undergraduate nursing university courses. As individuals are unable to understand others until they come to know themselves, self-awareness is a key element towards compassionate communication and emotional intelligence. Jack and Miller (2008) developed a self-development awareness tool for nurses by which they can recognise their strengths and limitations in the care they provide, clearly reflecting on their own acts and omissions.

Bailey et al. (2011) also developed a three-stage model, which illustrates how nurses learn to develop expertise in end-of-life care in the ED. Learning how to manage the potentially harmful influences of regular exposure to death experiences in the ED happens through multiple encounters with dying patients and their families, allowing HCPs to progress through these three stages. The first stage of the model is the 'Investment of the therapeutic self in the nurse–patient relationship', which can have a positive impact on the patient experience, by getting to know the patient better and by understánding their individual and holistic needs. At this stage, the development of this relationship could include a discovery of the patient's personal values and norms, expressed through their words, actions, and behaviours, and finding areas of 'shared values'. Focusing on the individual values could contribute to a more tailored holistic care provided to the patient. The second stage is 'Managing emotional labour in emergency work', which represents the progress from investing the self into the nurse–patient relationship, into handling the burden that comes with the grief and bereavement experienced through the death of that patient, the greatest obstacle at this stage being the distancing behaviour adopted as a measure of self-protection. At this stage, HCPs could incorporate in their practice coping measures, such as formal debriefs or informal conversations with colleagues or family members, that would contribute to successfully manage the burden of the death experience. These internal support services and adopted coping mechanism may have an even greater importance in successfully managing the emotional labour of the death experiences, in the light of the decreasing number of charities offering counselling services. The final stage 'Developing emotional intelligence' makes HCPs capable of solving problems, facilitate learning and manage change, having four principal components, such as self-awareness, self-management, social awareness, and relationship management. Development of training programmes that support preparation of HCPs for the various aspects of the death experience, and offering practical support, mentoring, and coaching for new starters, or for the less experienced colleagues, would allow a continuum in managing the death and dying experiences in the ED.

Another important element of education should incorporate cultural and social awareness surrounding death and bereavement. Similar to self-awareness, cultural and social awareness of death could be incorporated into the ED preceptorship programme, but also could form part of the undergraduate nursing studies. The modern Western societies, characterised by multiculturalism, could provide numerous opportunities to encounter acts of bereavement that are 'out of the ordinary' for someone raised in a westernised culture. Learning about and understanding the different cultural, ethnic, or social approaches to death and grief could help overcome several barriers faced by staff currently in the ED. However, training alone does not prepare staff for the realities of death and dying, only repeated exposure to this experience does. Developing end-of-life 'coaches' or 'mentors' in the ED, through an appropriate training course, would allow dedicated staff to provide support and assistance to those unexperienced with death, similar, to the support and guidance provided to students and newly qualified nurses. These roles would be similar to the 'nurse link roles' for various clinical conditions in the ED, or being an 'education link', a 'dementia champion', a 'practice supervisor', or 'practice assessor' in the department. 'Coaches' or 'mentors' could not only prepare new staff for this experience but could chaperone or shadow during shifts and have an active involvement in the 'after-event' support.

Support services for staff already exist in the ED, and participants in this study suggested they were effective, particularly the 'hot' and 'cold' debriefs, the TRIM support service, the informal conversations among colleagues, or the access to professional psychologists during the COVID-19 pandemic. However, many of these support services are self-directed and their usefulness greatly depends on the individual going through this experience (or the skills of those providing them, e.g., in leading a debrief session). 'Coaches' or 'mentors', as described earlier, could play a crucial role in overcoming these challenges, supporting HCPs in accessing these support services. Debriefing should be distinguished based on their purpose, into 'debriefing-to learn', also labelled as an after-event debriefing, and 'debriefing-to-treat', labelled as critical incident stress debriefing (Kolbe et al., 2021). The WHO (2012) recommends that psychological debriefs, such as the 'debriefing-to-treat' should not be used as an intervention method for people exposed recently to a traumatic event, as it will not prevent post-traumatic stress disorder, anxiety, or depressive symptoms. However, when a team may require coming together to promote a sense of control, understand recent events and support one another, an alternative method, the 'debrief-to-manage' is recommended, with the purpose to normalise reactions, without exploring in detail what happened.

Line managers could implement measures of understanding HCPs' individual values and norms, and the importance of these in relation to the care provided for patients, by incorporating these aspects in their formal and informal communication. Line managers during the induction, evaluation, and appraisal conversations could expand their appraisal and evaluation questionnaires to incorporate questions, and initiate conversation about everyone's personal values, yet also to investigate how these values shape staff's professional behaviour. Training those members of staff that line manage others in advanced communication skills should be part of the senior team's development plan in the ED. Similar questions or areas of investigations relating to personal values could be included in debrief protocols, evaluating the impact of each death case discussed on these forums. This individual evaluation of personal values will help managers offering better training and preparation for staff will help with a more balanced shift allocation and skill mix, yet will also support the change and improvement of the ED culture, becoming socially, culturally, and spiritually more inclusive.

Talking about the death experience was identified as the most preferred way of coping, therefore the development of a structured framework to conduct debriefs and a development of internal and external staff support network would be highly valuable. This could be developed as a research–practice collaboration to be undertaken through co-production with national organisations in the UK, such as NIHR ARCs (Applied Research Collaborations), Academic Health Science Networks and local organisations, such as SoAR (Southampton Academy of Research). These organisations could offer valuable resources and infrastructure to support this initiative. One of the aspects of standardising debriefs would relate to one of the findings of this study, the characteristics of cases which poses a higher threat to induce a negative impact on staff, such as sudden, unexpected, highly traumatic, or child and young adult deaths. Initiating a debrief after every such death in the ED for all participating staff, including a follow-up with the 'mentors' or 'coaches' and potentially some specialist services, could potentially minimise impact on HCPs. The acknowledgement of personal values, under these circumstances, would mean that the support provided for HCPs is not a 'one-size-fits-all', but it is tailored to individual needs and expectations.

The topics discussed in this book provide important considerations for policy-makers and organisations related to development of strategies, policies, and regulations to improve future provision of care. In the UK, current NICE guidelines focus on the provision of care for end-of-life patients and their families, such as the end-of-life care for adults – QS13 (NICE, 2011), end-of-life care for infants, children, and young people – QS160 (NICE, 2017a) or care of dying adults in the last days of life – QS144 (NICE, 2017b), and exclude provisions of wellbeing measures for HCPs exposed to the experience of death. Incorporating the findings of this study in developing new guidelines and policies would support the efforts of health service providers, not only to maintain and improve quality of care, but also to improve staff's job satisfaction, overall wellbeing, retention, and career progression. Setting realistic goals and objectives to change the culture of the ED, including policies, processes, and systems, can be challenging, time-consuming, those actively involved encounter numerous obstacles along the way, including overall pressures on the system generated by staff shortages, high number of patients entering the primary and secondary health services, lack of funding, or workforce strikes. While change can happen from the top, moving downwards, it is not impossible to generate change from the individual level, role modelling new behaviours and attitudes, encouraging others by showing a good example.

Changing the culture in the ED will require in my opinion three well-established steps:

1 **Defining the vision and benchmarks:**
   Implementation of an evidence-based practice requires well-established and clear benchmarks or measuring outcomes, measuring positive results, both in terms of patient care and safety, but also HCP's confidence and job satisfaction.
2 **Communicating objectives, celebrating successes:**
   Objectives, benchmarks, and outcomes need to be clearly and regularly communicated. Taking individuals onboard is only possible if goals are shared and tools are offered to accomplish these objectives. The positive impact these changes will have also needs to be communicated by line managers, ward managers, matrons, and care group managers and celebrated regularly on a department, a division, or organisation level. Communication can happen during meetings, handovers, huddles, using newsletters, social media, or any other internal electronic communication method. Communication needs to be a two-way process, allowing HCPs to give feedback or raise concerns.
3 **Transparency and accountability:**
   Transparency of objectives, processes, and benchmarks is needed to build trust. HCPs are more likely to accept and enact change they have had a role in bringing about changes, as opposed to change they feel has been forced on them. This is in turn more likely to be a factor in sustaining changes to practice along with someone being holding others accountable to the change, if there is a move to 'old habits and practice' returning.

While death is an objective reality, experiencing it, making sense of it, and dealing with its consequences on a personal level, remains a subjective encounter, influenced by a set of individual values and norms. Exposure to death, with adequate preparation and comprehensive support, can be an experience that will enable healthcare assistants, nurses, and doctors to become even more empathetic and compassionate towards their patients and their families, improve the provision of end-of-life care in the ED, and as such, fulfil the deeper meaning of their professional call, finding satisfaction and perspective in their careers.

Reference list

Bailey, C., Murphy, R., Porock, D. (2011). Professional tears: Developing emotional intelligence around death and dying in emergency work. *Journal of Clinical Nursing*, 20 (23–24), pp. 3364–3372.

Bailey, C., Orr, M., Hewison, A., Baernholdt, M. (2017). Learning about end-of-life care in nursing - A global classroom educational innovation. *Journal of Nursing Education*, 56(11), pp. 688–691.

Jack, K., Miller, E. (2008). Exploring self-awareness in mental health practice. *Nursing Standard*, 12(3), pp. 31–35.

Kolbe, M., Schmutz, S., Seelandt, J.C., Eppich, W.J., Schmutz, J.B. (2021). Team debriefings in healthcare: Aligning intention and impact. *British Medical Journal*, 374(2042). Available at: https://doi.org/10.1136/bmj.n2042 (Accessed: 03 March 2024)

Leadership Alliance for the Care of Dying People (2014). *One chance to get it right.* Available at: https://assets.publishing.service.gov.uk/government/uploads/system/uploads/attachment_data/file/323188/One_chance_to_get_it_right.pdf (Accessed: 04 September 2024).

NICE (2011). *End of life care for adults.* Available at: https://www.nice.org.uk/guidance/qs13 (Accessed: 04 September 2024).

NICE (2017a). *End of life care for infants, children and young people.* Available at: https://www.nice.org.uk/guidance/qs160 (Accessed: 04 September 2024).

NICE (2017b). *Care of dying adults in the last days of life.* Available at: https://www.nice.org.uk/guidance/QS144 (Accessed: 04 April 2024).

NICE (2018). *To develop new partnerships to achieve best practice in end-of-life care (EOLC) through the provision of education programmes.* Available at: https://www.nice.org.uk/sharedlearning/to-develop-new-partnerships-to-achieve-best-practice-in-end-of-life-care-eolc-through-the-provision-of-education-programmes (Accessed: 04 September 2022).

World Health Organization – WHO (2012). *Psychological debriefing in people exposed to a recent traumatic event. Recommendation(s) 2012.* Available at: https://www.who.int/teams/mental-health-and-substanceuse/treatment-care/mental-health-gap-action-programme/evidence-centre/other-significantemotional-and-medical-unexplained-somatic-complaints/psychological-debriefing-in-people-exposed-to-a-recent-traumatic-event (Accessed: 04 December 2024).

Index

Made in the USA
Monee, IL
12 November 2026

22aed9ac-a270-45e4-9bf9-2b98dee94c65R01